TRADITIONAL CHINESE MEDICINE

A Woman's Guide to Healing from Breast Cancer

TRADITIONAL CHINESE MEDICINE
A Woman's Guide to Healing from Breast Cancer

NAN LU, O.M.D., L.Ac.
with Ellen Schaplowsky

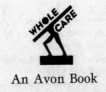

An Avon Book

The material in this book is for educational purposes only. Since each person's circumstances are unique, the authors recommend that you consult a physician with respect to your particular symptoms or medical conditions. The use of this material is the sole responsibility of the user at her discretion. The authors and the publisher cannot be held responsible for any liability or risk, personal or otherwise, that is incurred as a consequence of the application of the content of this book.

AVON BOOKS, INC.
1350 Avenue of the Americas
New York, New York 10019

Copyright © 1999 by Nan Lu, O.M.D., L.Ac.
Cover illustration by Hal Just
Back cover author photograph by Jaime Phillips,
courtesy of the Eddy Foundation
Interior design by Rhea Braunstein
Published by arrangement with the author
Library of Congress Catalog Card Number: 99-94877
ISBN: 0-380-80902-8
www.avonbooks.com/wholecare

First WholeCare Printing: September 1999

WHOLECARE TRADEMARK REG. U.S. PAT. OFF. AND IN OTHER COUNTRIES, MARCA REGISTRADA, HECHO EN U.S.A.

Printed in the U.S.A.

OPM   10   9   8   7   6   5   4   3   2

To my many extraordinary masters who have gifted me with the deep knowledge and spirit of true healing.

To my family—my parents and sisters, my wife Ling Shou and my children, Christina and Alicia.

—Nan Lu

To Nan Lu for his extraordinary ability to create light wherever he goes; To my son Ian, my sister Pat, and brothers Michael, Tom, Jim, and Peter; To my extended family, dear friends and Qigong sisters and brothers.

—Ellen Schaplowsky

Contents

Foreword

*O*NE day, in desperation, I decided to treat myself to a massage—not as an indulgence, but as an antidote to some of the symptoms from an autoimmune condition that I had been struggling with for several years without any relief from Western medicine. I thought a quiet hour would at least help me feel better for a while. Little did I expect to be introduced to "energy work," something I had never heard of, nor did I expect to hear about traditional Chinese medicine (TCM as it is called) and a doctor and master named Nan Lu. Nine months later, I booked an appointment with this man who, I must admit, looked to me to be too young to be able to help my situation. Lucky for me I was wrong. That fateful meeting was more than six years ago. Not only did Dr. Lu become my doctor and Qigong (or energy) master and I his patient and student, but he has also become my good friend and I have become his partner in the mission of bringing traditional Chinese medicine into the Western world in a practical and practicable way. His most powerful healing work to date has been in the area of women's health—especially premenstrual syndrome (PMS), menopause, and breast cancer. Lucky for all of us that he cares so deeply for his patients and has decided to shoulder the immense responsibility of anchoring the remarkable knowledge, techniques, and tools of this ancient medical system for today's Western women!

Breast cancer statistics retain a shocking familiarity. This disease now represents the most frequently diagnosed cancer for women in the United States with more than 180,000 new cases yearly. Annually, breast cancer claims more than 46,000 of our grandmothers, mothers, sisters, aunts, nieces, friends, coworkers, and acquaintances. It touches each of us in some way. In the United States, women have a one in eight lifetime risk of developing this condition. After heart disease, breast cancer ranks as the second biggest killer of women.

Early detection through breast self-examination and mammograms has been reported to help reduce mortality rates in some age groups and these tools remain vital in the fight against breast cancer. Globally, there are various research studies attempting to prove conclusively that this exercise or that food can help prevent breast cancer. While science searches for answers to the cause of breast cancer, halfway around the world, the ancient holistic medical system of traditional Chinese medicine has had an understanding of the cause of cancer for several thousand years and the root cause of breast cancer for more than five hundred years.

Over the course of five thousand years, TCM has helped literally billions of people. As a Western woman, I was more than amazed when Dr. Lu told me that it was common practice in ancient times for patients not to pay TCM practitioners if they became ill. The reason? The doctor had not done his job of keeping his patient well and preventing health problems! Dr. Lu says there are places today in China where medicine is still practiced this way. To me this time-tested philosophical orientation and practice of prevention seems light-years ahead of modern medical thinking, although I believe the two systems are finding more commonalties every day. What I have come to

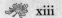

understand and deeply respect is that TCM is dedicated to helping the individual treat the source and not the symptoms of his or her problem. How simple this idea is, but how powerful.

Today, there are several billion people on this planet who think about health and healing in a way that is completely different from the way we think about them in Western society. Their thinking and experience has been shaped by this holistic, government-sponsored medical system that has been solidly in place and practiced continuously for more than five thousand years. This medical system, really a medical art, is based on the understanding of the human body as an ever-changing river of energy or Qi; it rests on the observation of living things rather than the dissection of dead ones. Its foundation lies with an unseen, yet real, force that is beyond science. Today, science is beginning to uncover many of the principles that ancient Chinese doctors have applied skillfully for centuries.

Many of us remember the Public Broadcasting System's landmark series, "Healing and the Mind," with Bill Moyers, which did much to introduce TCM and the self-healing energy practice of Qigong to a broad viewing audience in America. The event brought home the unusual power of TCM and its ability to produce with regularity what we might, in Western society, perceive as events that are miracle-like. This unique ability is not only the province of a few. For instance, Dr. Lu, with his master Professor Xi-hua Xu, demonstrated the power of Qigong at Fuzhou Hospital of TCM in 1995 with a group of women with breast masses. Their teaching of simple, ancient energy movements helped a number of these women reduce the size of their breast masses in just one session. Today in China, it is not uncommon to successfully treat breast cancer with Qigong; neither is it unusual to use a complementary program of Qigong, acupuncture, and herbal therapy with Western cancer treatments within the same hospital to give patients the best chance of healing from this devastating condition.

A wealth of TCM healing knowledge has been captured in this book. In my opinion, it is not an overstatement to say that this work constitutes a landmark effort. For the first time ever, it organizes and systematizes ancient self-healing knowledge that can help prevent breast cancer or breast cancer recurrences. Until now, Western women have never had access to this kind of comprehensive self-healing information that can help them in so many ways. We believe this TCM knowledge and its practical application as it is offered here can make a significant contribution to the fight against breast cancer.

This book is an important part of Dr. Lu's Breast Cancer Prevention Project, all parts of which are based on the ancient principles and theories of traditional Chinese medicine. The Breast Cancer Prevention Project also includes a practice video of the *Wu Ming* Qigong Meridian Therapy featured here, a website at www.breastcancer.com, and a series of *Wu Ming* Qigong workshops for breast and ovarian health. Some of these workshops, we are pleased to say, have been in conjunction with SHARE, the New York-based self-help organization for women with breast and ovarian cancer. In the future, Dr. Lu also plans to launch workshops for women suffering from menopausal side effects of the antiestrogenic agent tamoxifen. Over time, the Breast Cancer Prevention Project will include more self-healing programming and take its self-healing messages to women across the country and around the world. Everything in the Breast Cancer Prevention Project is based on TCM and its understanding of Qi, or vital energy, as some call it. As you read this book, you will learn a great deal about Qi. It is our hope that you will come away with a deeper perspective of how your body really works and the essential role Qi plays in maintaining a healthy body. Because of his lifelong special training with well-known, well-respected Qigong masters in China, Dr. Lu is uniquely qualified to create and develop this energy-based program. He is a high-level energy healer and his mission is to bring the benefits of this ancient healing system into Western society. (Additional information on Dr. Lu and his work can be found in the back of the book.)

In his gentle, wry way, Dr. Lu likes to remind his patients and Qigong students that TCM is not "New Age" medicine; nor, he says, is it a patchwork of different healing modalities. He likes to emphasize that TCM is a complete time-tested medical system—the only one that has identified a theory-based root cause for breast cancer. Why is this so important? Once the root cause is known, then specific treatments can be applied. Such is the case with TCM whose work on breast cancer began at least five centuries ago.

Today, Dr. Lu's own TCM practice focuses almost exclusively on Western women and helping them prevent illness and disease. He has treated many with a broad range of female health problems, but his attention is directed mainly toward women with PMS, menstrual irregularities, menopause, and now, breast cancer. Occasionally, I will see him shaking his head in disbelief that we Western women are so programmed to accept or cover up our female problems (which, from his perspective, are symptoms of much deeper and potentially more serious health issues) with continual medication. Dr. Lu's experience with his Western patients, coupled with his unique understanding of how to apply classical Chinese medical knowledge to help them, has led him to this point. There are many interesting examples of how he has applied classical TCM treatments throughout this book. Most important are his assessments and diagnoses of symptoms that relate to fertile conditions for the formation of breast cancer. I urge you to study the chart in Chapter 3 that outlines the Eastern and Western understanding of breast cancer's progression. You may be surprised at the information given for the early stages. In fact, you may see yourself and some current health conditions reflected there. These are conditions many Western women dismiss as insignificant or annoying. Or, they have been persuaded to believe that continual or periodic over-the-counter medication will banish their seemingly minor health problems. In some cases, we believe what you don't know *will* hurt you!

What is so wonderful about TCM springs from a fundamental understanding that we are all born with the ability to heal ourselves. This book offers the first comprehensive, natural, self-healing treatment program based on the principles and theories of TCM for women who want to:

- ✦ prevent a recurrence of breast cancer;

- ✦ relieve the side effects of chemotherapy, radiation, and tamoxifen;

- ✦ build up healing energy to successfully complete cancer treatment;

- ✦ reduce the risk of noncancerous breast tumors from becoming cancerous;

- ✦ address a range of female conditions, which TCM considers early warning signs of imbalances leading to breast cancer.

If you've already been treated for breast cancer (no matter what stage, no matter what combination of treatments), there is the sobering possibility it may come back. Without an understanding of the root cause of your breast cancer and why it occurred, only the symptoms can be treated. Currently in the West, there is no definitive information based on medical theory that pinpoints the root cause of breast cancer. Nor is there a comprehensive prevention program that goes beyond breast self-examination to help prevent breast cancer from occurring or recurring. Even the American Cancer Society states, "To date, knowledge about risk factors has not translated into practical ways to prevent breast cancer" (*Cancer Facts & Figures 1997*). While breast cancer treatments are increasingly more effective in attacking the disease itself, we believe that the ancient self-healing knowledge offered in this book adds a vital dimension of understanding to this issue by revealing its root cause.

Traditional Chinese Medicine: A Woman's Guide to Healing from Breast Cancer holds many benefits for the intelligent woman who wants to take responsibility for her health and believes that dynamic self-healing abilities reside within her body. Very simply, this book is for the woman who wants to take charge of saving her own life. It was fate that led me to Dr. Lu. I am deeply grateful to him for doing what the best ancient doctors did: help me unlock my own healing ability. It is fate that this book is now in your hands. It is a privilege and a pleasure to introduce Dr. Lu's unique work to you.

ELLEN SCHAPLOWSKY
Vice President
Traditional Chinese Medicine World Foundation

Introduction

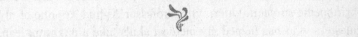

As a little boy in Fujian, China, I suffered from asthma. Because both of my grandfathers were doctors of traditional Chinese medicine (TCM), my condition naturally received a lot of attention. My father (a strong believer in TCM himself and an even stronger believer in the power of Qigong, China's ancient self-healing energy system) decided to put me under the guidance of a martial arts teacher. His hope was that this internal energy or Qi practice would help me strengthen my own healing ability. As time went on, I did heal and the asthma disappeared. I also came to love the martial arts, especially Taiji. I loved its philosophy, its movements, and the way it helped connect me to new levels of reality.

As a teenager, I was privileged to win the gold medal in the All South China International Martial Arts Competition. During my teen years, I competed often. I met many masters, some of whom imparted amazing gifts to me. Later, when I came to America, I realized that a lot of the things I saw and did, which I took for granted, are not only uncommon in a Western society, but are often looked at as "miracles." For instance, in martial arts competitions, where broken bones are an everyday occur-rence, it is not unusual for a doctor of TCM to set a simple break with herbal compounds, wrap it loosely (casts are hardly ever used), and give herbs to help boost Qi and blood circulation. Often, the injury heals in days. I've witnessed this many times, especially under the tutelage of the late Master Wan Laisheng, a well-known and very well-respected martial artist and orthopedic surgeon. Later, with Professor Xi-hua Xu, one of my masters who has helped my medical skills take a quantum leap, I saw the power of TCM in a hospital clinic in China with women who were able to reduce the size of their breast masses with Qigong in a single session.

These experiences and others helped me realize that authentic TCM could make a major contribution to health and healing (especially in the West) if its principles and theories could be presented properly and understood. This basically has become my challenge and my mission.

As a doctor of TCM, my own understanding of the need to help people learn about their self-healing abilities is continually reinforced by experiences with my Western patients. No matter which medical condition they suffer from, they usually arrive at my office as a last resort. Often they've traveled down just about every conceivable medical avenue to address their particular health problem or condition. I can tell they've reached the end of their line. Trying something unknown like TCM is often an act of sheer desperation.

Many of my patients have another experience in common: while they are suffering, often seriously, their scientific medical tests are considered normal. This complicates their physical and emotional conditions because it adds frustration on top of discomfort or pain. I feel very deeply for these people. Often, I am happy because I know TCM can offer them hope. What I can tell them is that, from the TCM perspective, their health problems are due to a Qi (vital energy) dysfunction or disorder. I can also tell them their current condition is beyond the realm of

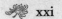

scientific testing, and has the potential of turning into a serious physical problem.

Using a simple analogy, I tell them: "Your body is like a car. All the parts are there, but to make the car run smoothly, you need gas and other functional fluids to keep it working. Today's cars have a warning light to let you know when you need more gas, or more energy. Our bodies also need 'gas' or energy to run well; we, too, have 'warning lights' that let us know when our energy is running dangerously low." We just don't know how to read these signs. Many of the physical and emotional symptoms that we think are systemic illnesses are really warning signs of a deeper problem. They tell us that our organs are not functioning well energetically or are not communicating with each other. In other words, they have a Qi or energy function disorder. (Here's another way to look at this: the body is also like a computer; it has developed a software problem, not a hardware problem.) TCM is a medical system whose foundation is built on the concept of Qi as the organizing force. TCM goes beyond the physical world to look deeply into the web of life that reflects how our bodies really work. It offers an ancient "blueprint" of your energy body and the means to keep it well.

I have worked with thousands of patients, about 90 percent of whom are women. What has affected me so deeply about the women that I care for is the suffering that they have undergone, often unnecessarily. For me this is very sad, especially when TCM treatments—acupuncture, acupressure, moxibustion, Qigong, herbs and food—can address the root cause of their problems. I have been especially moved by the dilemma of my Western women patients who are undergoing cancer (breast, uterine, and other) treatments. From my perspective, they have so little healing help while traveling this lonely and traumatic path. I feel it is my responsibility to help them, and now others, unlock their innate healing ability. I try to do this with every patient to the best of my ability.

There are many reasons I've taken on an effort as big as I hope the Breast Cancer Prevention Project will be. I am committed to educating all women that there are natural and effective healing actions they can take to help prevent breast cancer, as well as prevent a recurrence. And even if breast cancer develops, it is my belief these women will have less suffering than their counterparts who do not have the benefit of this self-healing knowledge. Watching my own patients and seeing their emotional, mental, spiritual, and physical struggles, as well as their successes, has given me the strength and the courage to launch such an undertaking.

Much of the suffering I witness, I am sorry to say, is not necessary. Many of the health problems of the women I treat are rooted in emotional conditions and related to their highly stressed lifestyles. From the TCM perspective, stress can actually be deadly. In TCM, five specific emotions are linked to the body's five major organ systems. Chronic stress and negative emotions are the strongest triggers of the lethal conditions that lead to breast cancer. You'll learn more about this when we get to a discussion of the liver. (This, incidentally, is not my opinion, but one expressed in a body of TCM work that goes back five hundred of its five thousand years!) As often as I can, I tell my patients to mind their hearts first, then mind their bodies. Thoughts are far more powerful than the body. What you think and feel has tremendous consequences for any disease, but especially breast cancer. Because Western women carry such heavy physical and emotional burdens, it is not surprising that the highest rates of breast cancer are found in Western countries (more than 100 cases per 100,000 women), while the lowest are in Asian countries (10 to 15 cases per 100,000 women). I fully expect, however, the rates in the East to increase as lifestyles there speed up and become more Westernized.

If we can widely communicate the information in the Breast Cancer Prevention Project and this book, then I believe women will have the opportunity and the tools to help themselves prevent breast cancer or its recurrence. When I understood that breast self-examination is considered the most important preventive tool Western women have, I became committed to helping them understand that there are so many more things they can do to avoid breast cancer that go far beyond breast self-examination. I believe self-examination and mammograms are important, but I regard them as early detection, certainly not prevention.

I am also committed to showing women the offensive way to address breast cancer. As essential as early detection is, waiting for a lump to appear is not true prevention. TCM has extensive experience in treating the root cause of breast problems. It is a fully realized medical system with sophisticated theories, techniques, and treatments successfully practiced for more than five millennia with hundreds of millions of people. So many Chinese women have benefited from TCM; now you have an opportunity to do the same. Beyond science, its foundation is the understanding of our body as an inseparable energy system with its parts in constant communication with all other parts, and this whole system woven into the much larger external Universe. I want to educate as many people as possible that TCM is not a random collection of treatment options, single herbs, or visualization techniques. It is a complete modality that takes into account the whole person—her body, mind, emotions, and spirit. Each of these aspects of the self must be carefully nurtured in the life and death struggle with breast cancer.

From everything I've experienced, everything I've learned, everything I know, and everything I believe, the ancient self-healing techniques of traditional Chinese medicine can make a major contribution to women in their fight against breast cancer. My Western women patients have taught me many, many things. Most importantly, they have shown me their desire and willingness to take responsibility for their own healing and work for it. It is my hope that passing along this ancient self-healing knowledge will help many more women help themselves through the journey that is breast cancer. This is my mission; this is my passion.

NAN LU

TRADITIONAL CHINESE MEDICINE
A Woman's Guide to Healing from Breast Cancer

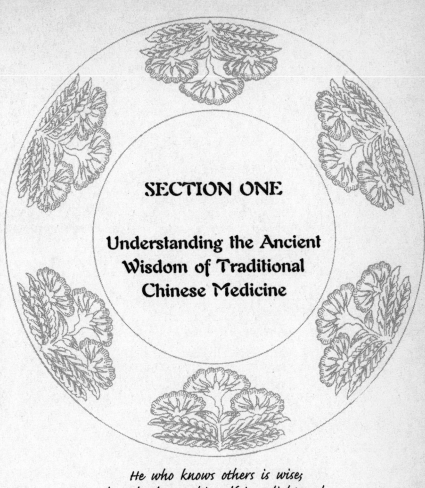

SECTION ONE

Understanding the Ancient Wisdom of Traditional Chinese Medicine

He who knows others is wise;
he who knows himself is enlightened.

He who controls others is powerful;
he who masters himself is beyond power;

He who enjoys his own reality is rich;

He who has a strong will is resolute;

He who follows his own nature endures;

He who follows the Tao has immortality.

TAO TE CHING (circa 500-200 B.C.)

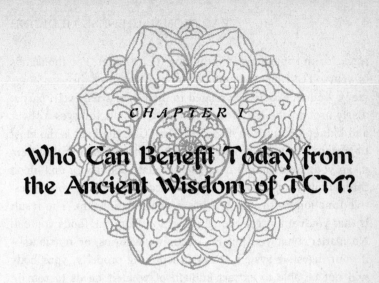

CHAPTER 1

Who Can Benefit Today from the Ancient Wisdom of TCM?

Traditional Chinese medicine (TCM) can support you during every stage of breast cancer, from the moment of diagnosis; to before, during, and after surgery; through chemotherapy and radiation; as well as during tamoxifen therapy. Perhaps most importantly, it has a wealth of sound advice for the healing journey you must take after completing treatment. TCM provides a comprehensive framework for dealing with the things you must change if you want to prevent cancer's energy pattern from taking hold again. Thousands of years ago, TCM theory stated that as long as Qi—internal vital energy—remains strong and flows freely and the body's organs work in harmony, disease or illness cannot enter. In other words, the answers to a healthy body lie inside your body itself. Your miraculous energy blueprint holds the key to true healing.

Whether or not you develop breast cancer, or experience a recurrence of breast cancer, depends on how strong your immune system is, how well your organs work together in harmony, and how well you take care of yourself. TCM believes there is always something you can do to help break this disease's energy pattern, whether it is controlling it, preventing its recurrence, or in some cases, eliminating it altogether. For thousands of years, TCM has understood the root cause of the symptoms many women experience related to their menstrual cycle, particularly around the age of menopause, and their linkages to liver and kidney Qi function disorders. (In TCM, the liver is the most important organ for women's health.) These function disorders mean your liver cannot help you circulate enough Qi and blood throughout your body and therefore cannot support your digestive function, with which it has a vital relationship. The result is that you cannot get enough nutrition from the foods you eat. No matter what you put in—vitamins, calories, or nutrients— if your digestive system is not functioning properly, your body will not be able to extract enough of what it needs to remain strong. As we shall see, this is especially relevant to women undergoing breast cancer treatment.

An energy disorder of the kidney means that the Qi, or life force, of this organ is too weak to function well and provide the right messages and power you need for the activities of everyday life. In other words, your engine is running poorly. Kidney Qi directly influences the health of the hair, the bones, and the body's overall Qi. This is why hair loss and general fatigue affect so many women undergoing energy-destroying breast cancer treatments. Unfortunately, these women have often depleted their kidney Qi through unbalanced and unhealthy lifestyle choices long before they reach the breast cancer treatment stage. These treatments then aggravate their underlying kidney Qi imbalance. TCM has treated patients with kidney Qi disorders naturally and effectively for centuries.

Today in China, many hospitals routinely use TCM therapies in conjunction with Western cancer treatments. The traditional Chinese medical system has had the support of the Chinese government for many centuries. Virtually all hospitals have a department of TCM, even hospitals that offer Western treatments. Both Eastern and Western practitioners in China understand and respect the fact that the TCM medical system is skilled at treating women during various stages of breast cancer and beyond.

Recently, the antiestrogenic agent tamoxifen has been introduced into breast cancer treatment regimens. Women who have been through surgery, chemotherapy, radiation, or a combination of treatments, and are taking tamoxifen, already have weakened digestive systems. Premenopausal women who have undergone chemotherapy and are taking tamoxifen may also experience a range of menopausal symptoms such as hot flashes, stomach distention, night sweats, constipation, insomnia, heart palpitations, hair loss, dry skin, vaginal dryness, loss of sexual desire, and the like. TCM has effectively treated these kinds of symptoms for thousands of years and can offer real relief in this area. Why do I call these conditions symptoms? We shall see that they are the result of problems or dysfunctions of an organ or organs. Possibly most important, TCM treatments are considered very effective in helping regenerate the immune system so that the patient remains strong enough to complete her breast cancer treatment. It accomplishes this with unique herbal formulas that can increase T cell counts between cancer treatments.

TCM takes a serious interest in a variety of women's health problems that Western medicine may view as routine at best, or may dismiss at worst. Please study the breast cancer progression chart in Chapter 3. This TCM perspective on the root cause and stages of breast cancer has never before been organized and published in the West or East. It looks at how the body and its systems weaken over time and progress toward breast cancer. The length of time that it takes to reach the final stage depends on the condition of each individual's Qi. (Many Western doctors believe that most cancers are in the body eight to ten years before detection.) Let's look at the implications of this:

1. If you already have a noncancerous breast tumor, or you suffer from breast tenderness, especially during your period, then according to TCM theory, your condition has progressed from a Qi function disorder to a physical problem. Generally speaking, your liver function has become unbalanced and is causing a serious problem. It is also possible that other organs have become unbalanced as well and are contributing to the cause of this breast tumor.

TCM can diagnose which organ has a function disorder from the location of the breast tumor. It can also diagnose Qi or energy blockages from reading your pulses and evaluating other warning signals from your body. (You'll find a list of warning signs to which you should always pay attention in Chapter 8. Please be sure and check to see if you have any.) It is possible to use the ancient wisdom of TCM in this book to restore internal harmony among your five major organs and help Qi flow unobstructed through your meridians. When this stage of good health is reached, TCM states there is no place for disease or illness to enter.

2. If your Qi function disorder progresses further, you become more at risk for breast cancer. At this point, however, your body still has the ability to restore normal function to your organs. Now is the time to help yourself naturally by following the Nine-Point Guide to Self-Healing outlined in Chapter 4. The most important step is the *Wu Ming* Meridian Therapy, ancient self-healing energy movements that can help your body's organs function in harmony again and help you avoid cancer's energy pattern. I cannot stress enough how much these movements can help you. Chapter 16 is the most important chapter in this book. For those predisposed to breast cancer through genetics or heredity, you know you are also at risk, particularly if you already have a breast mass. If your mass has not progressed to cancer, this means your body's Qi is still strong enough to fight with and control cancer's energy pattern. If, for any reason—let's say because of continual stress or chronic anger, or a catastrophic illness—your immune system collapses and your organs experience a function disorder, then cancer's energy can become powerful enough to overwhelm your own self-healing ability. If you can begin to understand cancer from the TCM perspective, you can then see how you actually have the power to stay in control of your own good health. This relates to the TCM theory of "yin and yang" energies, which we'll discuss in much more detail in Chapter 6. Again, the answer does not lie in the gene itself, but in the condition of your body. You yourself, even with a genetic predisposition, have the power to control whether or not this internal seed becomes cancer. Before this happens, use the ancient wisdom, techniques, and tools here and learn how to help yourself.

If you are affected by breast cancer, it is my wish that the knowledge provided here offers you hope, a sense of renewal, and the excitement of empowerment. One of TCM's most important principles states that each of us is born with the ability to heal ourselves. This gift never goes away; sometimes, however, we need help to reawaken its power. It is also my wish that traditional Chinese medicine will help you restore your unique healing gift.

The information in this book can help support women:

❧ Undergoing breast cancer treatments who are seeking natural ways to relieve their side effects and to prevent a recurrence of cancer in the breast or other areas of the body;

❧ Diagnosed with a nonmalignant breast tumor who are seeking natural ways to treat or control it;

✿ Seeking natural, self-healing methods that can help protect them from developing breast cancer.

TCM, its principles, theories, and successes are becoming more familiar to Western health-seekers every day. Qi, the foundation of TCM, is a concept that is gaining increased awareness and understanding in the West, thanks to the "Healing and the Mind" television series mentioned earlier, the work of the National Center for Complementary and Alternative Medicine (NCCAM) of the National Institutes of Health (NIH), which has recently accepted the efficacy of acupuncture for certain medical conditions, as well as the work of some of America's most respected universities, doctors, scientists, physicists and researchers. Before we move forward, let's take a look at some remarkable historical achievements in TCM.

CHAPTER 2

History of TCM and Its Understanding of Cancer

*J*ust how old the healing art of TCM is, no one really knows. Its true origins occurred long before its principles and theories were categorized and written down in the *Nei Jing,* the first TCM medical canon attributed to the Yellow Emperor. In the great global apothecary of indigenous medical systems, TCM is generally considered among the oldest in the world. And, while there are many great healing traditions, none is like TCM, which can claim that it has been in continuous practice with a government-sponsored system of practitioners, colleges and academies for more than five thousand years.

As we've said, TCM is deeply rooted in the understanding of Qi, the life force that animates all things. The theories and practices of TCM are a reflection of its profound connection to the natural laws of the Universe. Most people in modern society have no idea what "natural laws" are; however, these laws have a critical effect on health and healing. Whether an individual believes in them or not, when he or she tries to go against the "natural laws"—the invisible, real rules of the Universe—they become sick in either a minor or a major way.

Let's go into this a little more deeply. TCM believes that

the human body is a microcosm of the Universe—"as above so below." While your body must follow its own internal natural laws, it must follow Universal law as well. What does this mean in real life? For instance, it is a natural law that different seasonal energies are related to different organs. This is not a man-made concept. The ancient Chinese were able to receive and understand these concepts. They then passed them down for millennia. (These relationships are outlined in the Five Element Theory chart on page 84.) These different seasonal energies greatly influence their related organ's function.

Here's an example: TCM relates spring to the liver. If your liver does not function properly (that is, follow its own natural law), when the energy of spring arrives you will experience problems such as headaches, high blood pressure, emotional swings, excessive angry feelings, tendon problems, and even problems with digestion. In the case of a woman's breast, the liver and stomach are the two most important organs controlling its health. Here again, the natural laws are at work. If you're under great stress and suffer from chronic anger, you may experience breast tenderness, or even feel a breast mass during your menstrual cycle. Why? Because anger and stress are the two exact internal and external emotions that have the capacity to damage liver function. If you really want to fix the problem of breast tenderness, or even a breast mass, you must go to the source and rebalance the liver's function. TCM understands this connection as part of the natural law.

Natural laws are basically "the way things work" in reality. Everything has a connection and everything has an effect on every other thing. We are all truly woven together into the fabric of the Universe. This is why TCM practitioners can look at the whole body and its organ systems as one intricate feed-back unit. They know that according to natural law, the body's internal systems must first work in and of themselves. They then must function in harmony with the rest of the body's internal systems so that the entire organism functions well. Within this state lies good health. Today, modern science has developed a similar concept known as "whole systems theory," which encompasses the idea of extensive multiple feedback loops that provide vital information on the state of the entire system.

As I've mentioned above, the earliest extant classical Chinese medical text is the *Nei Jing,* written some twenty-five hundred years ago. This comprehensive work outlines the entire structure of traditional Chinese medicine and how it should be practiced. To this day, the *Nei Jing* and its philosophical, theoretical, and practical information form the foundation and the backbone of all TCM. It is a remarkable collection of material that summarizes and systematizes the concepts and theories of this ancient medicine. It describes in sharp detail the human body, how it works, the role of Qi and the meridians (the energy pathways that carry Qi throughout the body), as well as how the body interrelates with the spirit, the natural environment, and the greater Universe. It also addresses methods of diagnosis and treatment. Most importantly, it describes the principle of prevention. Prevention is TCM's specialty. The *Nei Jing* also provides the framework that allows TCM to treat the source and not the symptoms of illness and disease. To this day, the basic principles and theories in the *Nei Jing* have never been overturned or altered. This extraordinary work is also the first classical medical text to describe cancer, as well as specific cancers such as stomach, large intestine, and uterine. It also talks about the root causes of cancerous conditions. For example, the *Nei Jing* says uterine cancer can result "when the emotions of happiness and anger are out of balance . . . it can also develop when the body cannot adjust to environmental changes of cold and hot. If either or both of these conditions are present, then illness or unbalanced Qi can remain within the body where it eventually coagulates and forms a physical lump." This is the earliest reference to Qi stagnation and emotional imbalances as serious root causes of cancerous conditions.

The earliest Chinese medical reference to breast masses or tumors occurred during the Sui Dynasty (581–618 A.D.) in the *Zhu Bing Yuan Hou Lun* by Dr. Yuan Fang Chao. Dr. Chao describes a breast mass as ". . . a tiny lump that stays in the breast. This mass is not too hard and also not too big. Its shape is like a small irregularly formed stone." During the fourteenth century, a very famous Chinese physician, Dr. Dan Qi Zhu (1281–1358 A.D.), based his own theories on the work of the *Nei Jing*. His *Dan Qi Xin Fa* discusses breast cancer this way: "Because the wife does not enjoy a good relationship with her husband, nor does she enjoy good relationships with family members and others, then chronic anger, depression, worry and nervousness will accumulate in her day by day. This condition, if left unchecked, will cause a spleen Qi or 'digestive system' disorder, as well as liver Qi stagnation. Eventually, this will cause a small lump within the breast that causes no pain and no itchiness. Many years later, this lump will turn into a different shape (much like a craggy rock with many holes), which is called '*yan*,' or cancer. If the lump takes on this shape, it is very difficult to fix."

And, more than five hundred years ago, another TCM doctor outlined the root cause of breast cancer. Around 1400 A.D., Dr. Chen in his *Wai Ke Zhang Zong* stated: "These [negative] emotions accumulate day by day and cause spleen and stomach Qi deficiency and liver Qi stagnation. These conditions will cause the body to create a lump. When Qi or energy stagnates in the meridians over time, a small seed can progress to a cancerous mass. Then the five major organs will spiral out of balance. This problem is called breast cancer."

The *Nei Jing* gave TCM its form and structure. The theories and practices of this unique work have remained unchallenged for more than two thousand years. Over time, this body of healing knowledge expanded and, over the centuries, doctors of TCM made great strides producing many additional valuable medical texts that are consulted to this day. For example, in the third century A.D., Huang Fumi compiled the important work, *Zhen Jiu Jia Yi Jing*, from three previous works. It is the earliest comprehensive classical work on acupuncture and moxibustion (the application of heat to acupoints). In it, he outlines 349 acupoint locations on the body, their therapeutic properties and contraindications, as well as methods of needle manipulation. This book exerted enormous influence on the spread of Chinese medicine throughout the world. By 300 A.D., a medical text with more than 262 prescriptions for various diseases had also been written. This body of work basically laid the foundation for Chinese clinical medicine and formed the foundation of herbal prescriptions taught to this day in TCM colleges and hospitals throughout China.

Dr. Hua Tuen (b. 208 A.D.) is another illustrious TCM practitioner of the third century. Dr. Tuen is acknowledged as the first Chinese doctor to perform orthopedic surgery and understand the need for Qi to move through the body to accelerate recovery. He created a well-known series of Qigong movements for healing, which he adapted from observing the movements of various animals. Today in parks all over China, hundreds of thousands still practice this popular form of Qigong known as *Wu Qin Xi*.

Also somewhere in the third century, a book called the *Shen Nong Ben Cao (The Herbal)* came into being. It is the earliest extant classical text on "materia medica" handed down from this time. It summarizes the then known Chinese pharmaceutical knowledge, detailing more than 365 kinds of drugs and pharmacological theories. Interestingly, many of these have proven extremely valuable to modern clinical practice. For example, it recommends Chinese ephedra for asthma; goldenthread for dysentery, and kelp for goiter, among others. In identifying these herbal substances, doctors of TCM were recognizing not their scientific properties, but their Qi or energy properties.

Ancient doctors had the extraordinary insight and sensitivity to understand which herbs could enter specific meridians for healing purposes. Today, through TCM, we still have access to this unique body of knowledge. I have incorporated much of it in Chapter 17 in the list of classical herbs and herbal recipes that TCM uses for healing breast cancer. It is my privilege to present this information, because it has never been organized and presented this way—either in the East or West.

In the fourth century, Zhang Zhongjing's famous *Shang Han Lun* told how disease progresses, the best way to treat its various stages, the specific times of the day and seasons that are best for treatment, and how to stop disease. This is the earliest ancestor of all other books on the study of herbal prescriptions. Its specific formulas are used to this day both in China and around the world.

TCM has made many early and valuable contributions to the world's medical knowledge. For instance, it is credited with identifying parasitic infections as coming from a poor diet and the problems associated with eating raw meat. The ancient Chinese medical profession produced sophisticated works of pharmacology, understood the spread of disease through noxious air and water, and created extensive medical works on surgery. In the eleventh century A.D., long before Christopher Columbus had reached the New World, the Chinese had become pioneers in immunology with their work in the treatment of smallpox. They also correctly identified how disease is spread through the air and helped develop some of the earliest theories of epidemiology. Until this development, it was believed that illness or diseases could only enter the body through its surface.

TCM has had more than two thousand years of experience with cancer and at least five hundred years of experience with breast cancer. Its ancient assessment of the root cause of breast

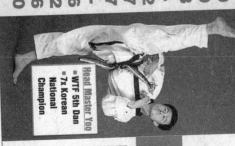

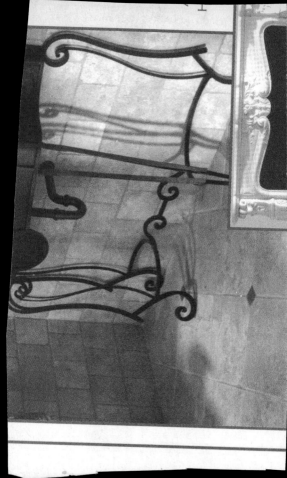

cancer is as valid today as it was in the distant past. Its approach has not changed, evolved or been altered. Even now, in cancer hospitals in China, TCM is used to complement Western breast cancer treatments to give women the best chance of healing. This ancient medical wisdom has helped millions of Chinese women. It is my goal to widely introduce this information in the West so that women can apply the best of Eastern and Western medicine to their own unique situation.

TCM is alive and well in China today. It is often used, with great effectiveness, side by side with Western medicine to treat a variety of diseases and illnesses. In some instances, TCM offers a significant advantage over Western medicine—especially in the treatment of chronic conditions or sports injuries. A nationwide government study done a decade ago in China discovered more than 40,000 practitioners; 1,500 hospitals with more than 100,000 beds; 26 colleges and 30 academies of traditional Chinese medicine.

In a recent meeting with Zonghan Zhu, M.D. of the Beijing Municipal Health Bureau and the World Health Organization (WHO) Collaborating Center for Epidemiology, I learned that 15 million permanent and temporary residents of Beijing are now being served by an increasing number of TCM hospitals. Dr. Zhu said that in the past ten years 18 TCM hospitals had been built at both the municipal and district or county level to better serve Beijing's population. He also told me that even general hospitals in China are required to set up a department of TCM and a pharmacy devoted to TCM classical formulas and herbs.

In China today, women have a choice when they go for breast cancer treatment. They can use Eastern or Western medicine, or a combination of both. When I ask my patients how they would treat their condition if they could go to the best American medical treatment centers or the best American hospitals and have a choice of combining natural healing methods with Western treatments, I am not surprised by their answers.

CHAPTER 3

East and West: A Story About the Root Cause and Progression of Breast Cancer

*I*F there is one single concept that I want you to take away from this book, it is that according to TCM theory, you absolutely cannot get cancer if your organs work in harmony and Qi flows freely throughout your body's meridian network. This theory has been practiced successfully by TCM doctors for thousands of years with millions of patients. It has not yet been proven by Western science, but parts of it have. To one degree or another, any woman who develops breast cancer has experienced one or more symptoms, which have worsened over time, that TCM can readily identify as Qi stagnation and/or an organ function disorder. The sad part of this is that the patient did not recognize them for what they were: early warning signs.

This TCM theory opens the door for you to understand how you can take full responsibility and control over your health to prevent or help heal breast cancer.

Rather than reacting to the monthly anxiety of cancer detection, you now have a comprehensive framework within which you can look positively at your whole body and the tools and techniques to apply its wisdom in your everyday life. If you have had or have breast cancer, this TCM theory will redirect your attention to its root cause. This can help you effectively destroy cancer's negative energy pattern and prevent its return.

Remember that detection is detection, not prevention. There are many, many small easy steps you can take today that cumulatively can help prevent a major health disaster tomorrow.

Once you understand the holistic TCM concept of treating the body, mind, and spirit, you can see why individual treatments like chemotherapy and radiation, or individual drugs, or individual supplements are only good for some people some of the time. The Western way is to treat the disease; the TCM way is to treat the whole person.

The chart on page 18 has never before been seen either in the East or the West. I have outlined, for the first time, a side-by-side comparison of the progression of breast cancer as it is understood by TCM and Western medicine. The easiest way to understand this chart is to use it to follow the health history of our composite patient, Mary Smith.

Mary is not unusual, but she is unique. She has been married for twenty years and is in her early forties. She has two children ages thirteen and fifteen. She works full time and runs a small division within a fast-growing communications company where she manages six people. Her mother lives in a nursing home, which she visits frequently, but not as often as she believes she should. In the fall, she is a "soccer mom." Mary is extremely busy and she always seems to be playing catch up with her life. At times, the stress of being a wife, mother, executive, caretaker, and volunteer seems overwhelming.

Every once in a while, Mary has a pretty bad headache right across her forehead. Sometimes her temples throb. She will take an aspirin or other pain reliever and take a rest. When she does this, her headaches disappear and she chalks them up to her overcommitted life: a promotion (a title, but no money), carpooling two teenagers, and her husband's new side business. If she mentions these occasional headaches to her Western doctor,

Progression of Breast Cancer According to TCM Principles

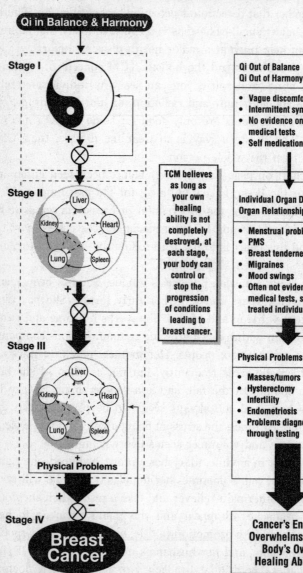

Qi in Balance & Harmony

Stage I

+ − ⊗

Qi Out of Balance
Qi Out of Harmony

- Vague discomforts
- Intermittent symptoms
- No evidence on medical tests
- Self medication

Stage II

Liver
Kidney — Heart
Lung — Spleen

+ − ⊗

TCM believes as long as your own healing ability is not completely destroyed, at each stage, your body can control or stop the progression of conditions leading to breast cancer.

Individual Organ Dysfunction/
Organ Relationship Problems

- Menstrual problems
- PMS
- Breast tenderness
- Migraines
- Mood swings
- Often not evident on medical tests, symptoms treated individually

Stage III

Liver
Kidney — Heart
Lung — Spleen
+
Physical Problems

Physical Problems

- Masses/tumors
- Hysterectomy
- Infertility
- Endometriosis
- Problems diagnosed through testing

+ − ⊗

Stage IV

Breast Cancer

Cancer's Energy
Overwhelms Your
Body's Own
Healing Ability

most likely she will not raise much interest because her head pains seemingly disappear on their own and all her tests are "normal."

However, if Mary goes to a TCM doctor at this stage, he or she would find her headaches very interesting, and something to explore further. The TCM practitioner would ask a number of general questions about these intermittent headaches. After a pulse diagnosis, he would ask Mary very detailed questions about them: Where are they located? What kind of pain do they produce—sharp, dull, aching, or needle-like? How severe are they? What time of day or night do they occur? Does weather aggravate or bring them on? Are they related to her period? The TCM doctor would question Mary as he or she had been taught—through the memorization of an ancient poem that tells what to ask of the patient. The TCM doctor's diagnosis? Mary's Qi is out of balance; she has a Qi, or energy, deficiency. (And, because these headaches occur across her forehead, the doctor knows immediately that her stomach is being affected.) Mary's Qi is not consistently strong enough to keep her five major organ systems working in harmony.

The TCM doctor would then tell Mary that the location of her headaches is important and that they are located precisely where the stomach meridian runs. This is an indication that her stomach meridian is affected. Mary tells the doctor her stomach is fine. This is considered Stage I. The TCM doctor would advise Mary that she should identify ways to change her lifestyle and that she should take better care of herself by resting and eating for healing. He would tell her to avoid all the cold foods and drinks she has been ingesting and switch to warm ones. He would also advise her that if certain things in her life do not change, sooner or later she can expect to experience more discomfort, possibly PMS, breast tenderness, vaginal discharge, or even the development of a breast mass.

It is about two years later and Mary's headaches are now

pronounced and more frequent. It is harder to get rid of them. They are now compounded by breast tenderness during her period. Sometimes Mary can feel a small mass during her period, but she is relieved that it disappears when she stops menstruating. She has developed PMS symptoms. And, although she cannot understand why, her stomach frequently feels distended; she has loose stools and seems to be allergic to foods she loves. She takes many pills to alleviate these worsening symptoms. Her Western doctors are sympathetic, but they tell her that her blood and other tests, such as a CAT scan, are "normal." They suggest a number of things to address her symptoms. They tell her they do not know why she has these symptoms or what is causing them and recommend several different prescriptions for the headaches and stomach problems, as well as for the side effect of the headache prescriptions.

If Mary goes to the TCM doctor at this point, he would advise her that she now has an organ function disorder. He would tell her that while the physical organ may still be all right, the way it works or functions is not. The doctor would spend time with Mary discussing her emotional condition. She would describe her anger about working too much overtime, which causes her to feel guilty about not seeing her mother in the nursing home enough. She would also tell him about the continual stress she's experiencing because her mother has just been diagnosed with Alzheimer's disease. The other things she's worried about is that she and her husband are faced with finding the funds to send their children to college, and they don't know where they're going to come from. It also doesn't help that she is under a lot of pressure at work and is not particularly close to any of her coworkers. Lately her anger seems constant and not as easily controllable as it was a few years ago.

In this case, using TCM theories, the doctor would now diagnose Mary with a liver function disorder. Her liver (the most important organ for women's health) is not functioning properly. The doctor would tell her that while her physical liver itself is all right, the way it works or functions is not. It's like a computer—the hardware is all right, but the software running the program is malfunctioning. The doctor would advise Mary she needs to be treated immediately with acupuncture and herbs. He would educate her about the root cause of her problems. He would discuss the need to go to the source to eliminate the problem. He would also advise her that if she continues taking pain killers and doesn't deal with the root cause, her condition could become even worse. This is now Stage II.

If Mary visits her Western doctor at this point, he will most likely order a number of scientific tests, including a CAT scan, blood tests and a check of her hormone levels. If all the test results come back normal, the doctor must conclude that she is well. He may empathize with her discomforts, but he now has no clues left to help him help her. He may prescribe different pain killers for her headaches. If her condition continues for a while and her tests remain normal, he may suggest she visit a psychologist. At Stage II, there are several reasons why Western medicine cannot understand the true source of Mary's physical discomforts: The most important reason is that Western medicine has no frame of reference for relating menstrual cycle headaches with liver function disorder; another reason is that there are no machines capable of testing Qi imbalances in specific organs. These conditions are beyond the realm of science.

With her TCM practitioner, Mary would receive immediate treatment. His treatment goal would be twofold: relieve her liver Qi stagnation (which can help her headaches and other physical symptoms) and prevent the liver function disorder from affecting her stomach further and reaching her kidney. Her TCM doctor would talk to her about how organs fall out of balance and how their communications with other organs becomes disrupted. Her doctor would also talk about the dangers of Qi stagnation in the meridians and how blocked Qi can eventually turn into matter and create a mass. He would also tell Mary that she is wearing herself out with her nonstop schedule and he is worried because he detects signs that her kidney Qi is declining. In this state it is very difficult to remain healthy. This could lead to a crisis where her whole body could become sick.

Let's move forward about another four years. Mary returns to her Western doctors. She has many more physical complaints. Most worrisome for her, this time she has discovered a small lump about one centimeter that does not go away. She is naturally alarmed. Her family doctor sends her to a cancer specialist who performs a biopsy. Mary feels very lucky because her lump is not cancerous. At this point, Mary has two choices: she can undergo a lumpectomy or she can wait for six months and be rechecked. The specialist sends her back to the family doctor to treat the headaches and other physical problems, which have never gone away.

If Mary revisits the TCM doctor, he would tell her that her problem has progressed to Stage III. It has gone from a Qi deficiency to a function disorder to a physical problem. She must treat this immediately with acupuncture and herbs to tackle the root cause. In addition to acupuncture, he would prescribe herbs that she can take internally and also give her an herbal powder to apply to her breast tumor to help shrink it. He would strongly urge Mary to change her lifestyle right away. He would tell her that her daily life is affecting her health. He would be particularly concerned about how she handles the constant stress she's under and worried that her anger and frustration has become chronic. He would tell her that continual stress and anger can have a deadly effect on her liver and that—without a lifestyle and emotional shift—she is in real danger of having her tumor suddenly take a quantum leap and become cancerous. If that happens, it would be very difficult to fix. All that this seed is waiting for is the right time and the right temperature to grow. If these conditions occur, there is no stopping its processing.

And the root cause, or cancerous seed, will live in her body until it is cut off completely.

Now, many of my patients ask me if stress directly causes cancer. I tell them that it is absolutely critical for women to understand that stress can cause a liver function disorder. When a woman has a liver function disorder, her blood and Qi can stagnate and cause a breach in her immune system. When this happens, she becomes vulnerable to breast cancer. Look what happens to Mary.

About six months later, she has a mammogram, and unfortunately, Mary is diagnosed with breast cancer.

TCM offers each patient hope. Take a look at the chart and note the feedback symbols on the TCM side. These relate to a very important principle. TCM believes that at each of the stages we've described, it is possible to control the progression of a health problem or fix it. This depends on the overall condition of the patient and the skill of the doctor. Stage I is usually easy to fix because the organs are still functioning in harmony. Stage II is somewhat more difficult because one or more organs are suffering from a dysfunction. This situation takes longer to help the body come back into balance. Stage III and IV are challenging even for the most skilled TCM doctor. But even at this point, TCM still believes that the condition can be controlled as long as the patient's own healing ability can be helped to refunction or rebalance itself.

In other words, TCM believes you can have breast cancer (or other cancer) for the rest of your life, but you won't die from it. I like to use this analogy when it comes to describing the TCM approach to treating breast cancer in its later stages: It's like having a bad tenant in your apartment building. He may not pay the rent, but as long as he doesn't bother the other tenants (affect other organs) or cause any problems, he can remain in the building. You can spend more energy kicking him out (with chemotherapy and radiation) than letting him stay.

The intelligent thing might just be to let the tenant remain and make sure he is contained and stays quiet and inactive. The TCM treatment approach is to increase the patient's energy foundation and strengthen her own healing ability to the point where it is strong enough to control cancer's energy and prevent its growth. This approach is not an uncommon choice for women in the East.

Part of the reason I wanted to write this book on breast cancer was to show women how and why breast cancer happens and how they can recognize early signs and certain conditions that, if left untreated, place them squarely on the road to this devastating disease. I also wanted the opportunity to provide women with a framework that allows them to understand the connections these kinds of health events have on the entire body. Otherwise, Western women particularly, have no way to put the many kinds of symptoms they experience into a meaningful context.

Here's an example I frequently use in my lectures to explain the importance of treating the source and not the symptoms of any health condition: When you drive your car and the indicator light for overheating comes on, what do you do? If you're like most sensible people, you immediately pull over to the side of the road. You know that if you continue to drive without taking care of this problem, you could ruin your engine. Let's assume you can get your car to a mechanic. He checks out your entire car and tells you it's fine, however, the indicator light is still glowing. If he tapes over the light, would you continue to drive this car? If he takes a hammer and smashes the light, would you feel comfortable driving this car? We all know that something inside the car is connected to this warning light. Just because the mechanic can't find a problem, doesn't mean there isn't one. Now reexamine our chart and look at Stage I or II. If you suffer from intermittent discomforts such as headaches, stomachaches, PMS, or menstrual irregularities, do you really think that the best course of action is covering up the symptoms with over-the-counter remedies? I must emphasize that the discomforts mentioned are not normal conditions for a healthy body. These symptoms are there for a reason. You will see that while breast self-examination and mammograms play a role in early detection, there is something beyond them that women can do for themselves to address the source of breast cancer.

Nine-Point Guide to Self-Healing: How to Use TCM Knowledge to Treat the Root Cause of Breast Cancer or Help Prevent It

$\mathcal{N}ow$ that you have some background on the skill of ancient TCM practitioners, I would like to share with you why and how authentic TCM works. When you understand its principles, theories, and techniques, you will be able to apply its power for your own healing protection against breast cancer. Let's start by reviewing the following Nine-Point Guide to Successful Self-Healing that I developed for my patients. It is based on the ancient understanding of the root cause of breast cancer and how to address it. If you would like to go into more detail about the root cause of breast cancer, go to Chapter 5 and then come back to this chapter.

Based on the TCM understanding of the root cause of breast cancer, there is no comprehensive medical theory-based program in the West that can help women prevent breast cancer or breast cancer recurrences. To date, no program, no organization, no hospital, no drug therapy, and no individual has offered an understanding of the root cause of breast cancer. In *Cancer Facts & Figures 1997,* the American Cancer Society stated, "To date, knowledge about risk factors has not translated into practical ways to prevent breast cancer. Since women may not be able to alter their personal risk factors, the best opportunity for reducing mortality is through early detection." TCM has a different view. From its perspective, there are a number of specific ways women can identify their personal risk factors and concrete steps they can take to address them before breast tumors or breast cancer appears. This knowledge is based on the experience and expertise derived from five hundred years of treating breast cancer's underlying causative factors.

As we have seen from the journey of our composite patient Mary Smith, there is no framework in the West for evaluating the many discomforts that women suffer in relationship to menstruation. These discomforts link their physical and emotional symptoms to serious early warning signals that they are becoming at risk for breast cancer. Our practical nine-point guide can be used to complement Western medicine. This material can also be used in conjunction with breast self-examination and early detection programs such as mammograms to give you the very best chance for good health and true healing.

Please take a moment to understand the following steps and use the wealth of TCM information in this book to change your life forever.

> *1.* Take inventory! Answer the questions in the six self-healing TCM checklists in Chapter 15 and test your level of knowledge about what can really harm or heal your body.

The self-healing checklists in this section relate to your lifestyle and daily habits. They cover eating, sleeping, work, pleasure, emotional conditions, and frequent discomforts. TCM understands that you can only have a healthy body if your daily life is in balance. I try to educate my patients that it is indeed the little things that count. Because TCM can treat the whole person and not the disease, it has identified which organ is related to what different condition. Often these conditions are related to lifestyle problems. These questions are based on TCM theories.

They are designed to help you have a better understanding of your lifestyle and your daily habits and how they may be damaging your physical health. You may be surprised at both the questions and the answers. The checklists will help you identify early warning conditions that could develop into more serious problems, if you don't take the time to address them now. The answers also reflect TCM theories.

> **2.** Learn the principles and theories of TCM and how the body, mind, and spirit work as a unit. Discover the secret of successful breast cancer healing and prevention that goes beyond breast self-examination—how to generate Qi, how to save Qi, and how to use Qi wisely. Qi, of course, being the very lifeforce that animates our physical bodies and everything else in the Universe!

Chapters 5 and 6 are very important. They provide an overview of the ancient principles and theories of TCM. Unlike Western science, where today's latest study is often contradicted by tomorrow's newest research, most TCM principles and theories have never been broken or challenged, let alone overturned. They have stood the test of time precisely because they reflect the natural law and a deep understanding of how the body really functions. These principles and theories have been in practice for many thousands of years and have traveled to many countries around the world. Untold millions of people have benefited from this unique holistic medical system. TCM specializes in treating the root cause of conditions—often, as we have seen, conditions that Western medicine has no framework for identifying, or if identified, cannot treat at the source. Because TCM does not treat the disease, but treats the individual as an organic whole, it can offer major improvement in certain chronic conditions such as arthritis, systemic lupus erythematosus (SLE), chronic fatigue, hypoglycemia, menopause, and many others that confound Western medicine. TCM also specializes in prevention, as well as in the art of sparking the individual's own healing ability. Its understanding of the properties and movement of Qi, or vital energy, goes far beyond science. Recent scientific developments are beginning to uncover and adapt these theories. For example, more than two thousand years ago, the *Nei Jing,* which characterized bone marrow as an "extra energy system," stated that "bone marrow can produce blood." In this light, today's focus on bone marrow by Western medicine is interesting.

    3. Practice *Wu Ming* Meridian Therapy for twenty minutes at least once a day.

The most important part of this book is the *Wu Ming* Meridian Therapy in Chapter 16. It is impossible to overemphasize the amazing benefits this ancient self-healing practice can bring you. There are seven, easy-to-perform energy movements that I have worked with my own master, Professor Xi-hua Xu, to adapt for breast health and breast problems. The entire program is designed to help unblock Qi in the meridians running through the breast area. These are not physical exercises, but meridian stretches. You can consider them a meridian tuneup. Practicing these movements helps you guide your own healing Qi. The first benefit is preventive in nature. It can help your five major organs function in harmony and jump start your own healing ability. The second benefit addresses Qi stagnation problems. Specific movements can help unblock Qi stagnation in specific organs or meridians. This seven-movement program of *Wu Ming* Meridian Therapy is the key to preventing breast cancer or its recurrence, and helping it heal. Daily practice can help change your life.

    4. Map out an "Eating for Healing" plan that incorporates as many healing foods and classical herbal recipes listed in Chapter 17 as possible.

Using foods to treat and heal various problems is one of TCM's special techniques. A very long time ago, TCM doctors were so attuned to energy that they could "see" the energies of foods and which organs they could benefit. Their insight went far beyond calories, vitamins, nutrition, and scientific properties. This knowledge has been passed down for thousands of years and is still valid and the prescription of foods is still in use. I have created a list of foods used by ancient TCM doctors and still prescribed to this day that can help the various organs involved with breast cancer. This is a very important list. Do not be fooled by the fact that these are common, everyday foods. Because of their essences and the Qi they carry, they can be powerful allies in helping boost your own Qi to fight or prevent breast cancer.

5. Learn how TCM herbs can help you stimulate your healing ability.

TCM has one of the oldest and most sophisticated herbal apothecaries in the world. The same energy principle applies to TCM's use of classical herbs as it does to its use of foods. These herbs and herbal formulas have been used, in many cases, for thousands of years. Today, scientific studies are proving that many of them have significant healing properties with regard to cancer and that they can strengthen the immune system between cancer treatments.

6. Look at where you spend your emotional energy and make the necessary changes that will save your life.

More than two thousand years ago, TCM recognized the powerful role emotions play in our health. Its practitioners knew that any excess or imbalances of the seven emotions (we'll discuss these more in depth in the following chapter) could cause disease or illness. Today, stress, which is one of the most destructive forces affecting the body, is everywhere. It is especially lethal for women because it affects the liver, which is the most important organ for women's health.

> **7.** Tap into nature's energy to support your own health and healing.

Whether you can feel it or not, whether you believe it or not, the human body is part of the larger Universe . . . Remember "as above, so below." If you can follow the natural cycle of things and tap into nature's pure energy, you can draw additional energy to remain healthy or help heal yourself. That's why taking a walk in the park or near the ocean is far more preferable than spending hours in the gym on a treadmill. One provides a living environment rich with energy's vibrations where you can connect with the healing power of nature; the other separates you from it.

> **8.** Chart your progress toward optimum health with the TCM self-healing evaluation form on page 322.

The questions in this self-healing evaluation form are based on the TCM theories outlined in this book. They are designed to help you identify the status of your own physical condition and where you might be out of balance. It may call attention to some symptoms you may not have noticed or given much attention to. It is very important to realize that these are related to early warning signs that could lead to the development of breast cancer. By practicing *Wu Ming* Meridian Therapy, your self-healing ability will gradually rebalance itself.

I have structured the knowledge in this book in such a way that you can use it to create your own self-healing routine. This routine can be especially beneficial if you have breast cancer, want to prevent a recurrence, or are serious about prevention. The first step is to make several copies of our self-healing evaluation form and periodically reexamine your physical condition and the symptoms you first noted.

Work with the TCM information in this book. Practice *Wu Ming* Meridian Therapy at least twenty minutes a day. If you can spend more time, that is even better. Review the special energy gates and begin a program of daily massage. Then, take time to read over the information about healing foods and herbs. Include as many of them that relate to your unbalanced symptoms as possible.

9. Continually send yourself the message that you are healthy and whole. Continually tell yourself that you intend to remain healed, or that you have already healed yourself— and believe it! Your mind is far more powerful than your body.

The Chinese believe that the mind can create "heaven or hell." Nothing is stronger than the thoughts you think. Your mind is superior to your body. It is vital to send yourself the most positive messages you can to remain healthy, or to recover from an illness like breast cancer. The purpose is to send a message to your internal self to re-awaken the healing ability you were born with. This type of mind practice is one type of Qigong where the practitioner uses her mental power to stimulate her body's defenses. Once the mind becomes stronger, the body's functions will follow. TCM says "*Yi tao; Qi tao.*" When the mind—*yi*—reaches a particular healing place, then the healing energy—*Qi*—will follow there.

I wish you success on your healing journey.

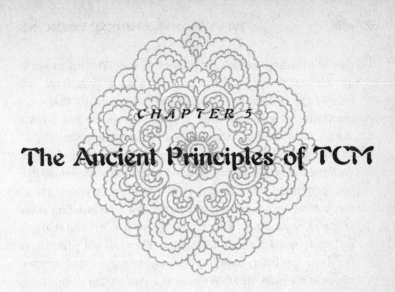

CHAPTER 5

The Ancient Principles of TCM

T_{CM} principles relate to the human body in a unique way. When it comes to breast cancer, I believe it is important to let Western women understand that these time-tested principles have worked for millions of Chinese women for millennia. When you come to a deeper understanding and appreciation of this ancient healing art, you too will be able to use its wisdom for your own self-healing. Acquiring this knowledge will also give you more control over your own health. Let's review the basic principles of TCM and some examples from my patients that provide insight into how these principles work.

❧**TCM believes that everyone is born with self-healing ability.**

TCM believes that at birth you are born with the ability to heal yourself, not just from minor things like a cold, but from major assaults on your system. You have all the chemicals, the neuron connections, messages ingrained in each organ, and the Qi or energy to get these messages from one organ to another in a smooth, efficient, and productive way. As we get older, many of us lose the ability to access this self-healing power, but it is never lost. The information always resides within the body. As long as you have two things: Qi, or vital energy, and five major organs that communicate at some level as a system, you always have a chance to make your healing ability function again.

Let's use your car as an example. If your battery is dead, you must replace it; but if it's low, there's a chance that you can jump start it and recharge it so it continues to work. Now let's take your computer. For it to function properly and be useful to you, it needs power (Qi), and it needs software in the form of a program. Then, all your hardware (keyboard, printer, monitor, etc.) must connect and communicate with each other. Without the power, the computer is useless; without the hardware and the software, it is nonfunctional. Both are essential. These simple analogies may help you understand how TCM regards the body and the things it needs to function in a healthy way.

The goal of this book is to introduce you to these concepts and help you learn how to recall your self-healing ability. I hope you will do this by creating your own healing program with the information offered here on energy movements, eating for healing, as well as daily changes for your body, mind and spirit that you can make to help heal yourself.

TCM believes that you must take responsibility for your own health and healing. I find many patients willing to do this, but they don't know where or how to begin. The ideal TCM doctor forms a partnership with the patient and helps the patient get in touch with her own healing abilities. TCM is a medicine of connections and interaction. In my practice, I work with my patient to create good communication so each of us can become sensitive to the subtle changes that will take place within her body. We want to be ready to respond when her self-healing spark is reignited; we want to nurture that spark into a full flame! I hope that through this book, we too can create a kind of partnership that will help you use your intuition to connect with this knowledge. Here are some interesting stories about some of my patients whose healing abilities were strong enough to overcome their problems with help from TCM. I remember one patient in her early thirties who had had heavy bleeding for a month. She tried many different things to stop this bleeding. Finally, her doctor recommended that she have a hysterectomy. (Hysterectomies are the most common operation in America for women in their forties.) Both she and her husband were very sad because they had hoped to have children. During her first appointment, I explained that from her pulse and tongue diagnosis, she had an energy or Qi deficiency coupled with liver Qi stagnation. I told her she would have to drink herbs (which are pretty terrible-tasting, I must admit), take a rest, and reduce the emotional levels and stress in her life. I told her we might be able to stop this bleeding in three or four days, if she could cooperate. She had reached the point where she would do almost anything to avoid a hysterectomy and agreed to commit herself to this course of healing. After four days, the bleeding stopped and she was able to save her uterus. It's important to emphasize that the treatment was not designed to stop the bleeding, which was a symptom (a serious one) rooted in a much deeper problem. I went after the source. I continued to work with this woman so that we could increase her overall Qi and relieve the liver stagnation so that this problem would not recur.

I had another patient who had a kidney stone. He too was desperate not to have an operation. After a pulse diagnosis, I found out his Qi, or vital energy, was still strong and that his organs were functioning pretty well. However, his kidney and bladder Qi were just not strong enough to naturally pass his kidney stone. I asked if he was willing to drink an herbal mixture that would help him boost his immune system immediately; he said he would. I then used acupuncture to increase his overall Qi and gave him enough herbs for one week. Within two days, he called me in amazement to say that he had passed this stone. Again, the treatment I prescribed was not designed to increase the amount of urination in the hopes of eliminating the kidney stone, rather it was to increase the Qi of the key organs involved so that his own body could take care of the problem naturally.

❧TCM believes that destructive energy patterns like cancer can be interrupted and broken.

TCM has a different concept of treating illness and disease. Viewing these conditions as negative energy patterns, TCM believes that destructive patterns like cancer can be interrupted or broken. Cancer is one kind of intelligent energy; it has another quality too—it is patient. It can wait in your body for many years without giving you a problem. This energetic force possesses the ability to analyze your body, figure out where to hide, and then stubbornly refuse to let go. Once you really understand this concept, you will understand why, if you have cancer or have had cancer, it is so important not to resume your old lifestyle. It is precisely your old lifestyle that provided a comfortable haven for this energy in the first place! You must learn how to let this negative energy go, and often with it the destructive habits that allowed it to remain in the first place. Again, I want to emphasize that the most important part of this book is the special ancient energy movements of *Wu Ming* Meridian Therapy in Chapter 16. They can actually help interrupt and break cancer's energy pattern by unlocking your body's own healing energy resources and directing them where they are needed. I also want you to learn how to change your energy pattern so that cancer can never find a comfortable home in your body again. Done on a daily basis, *Wu Ming* Meridian Therapy also provides a powerful prevention tool.

❧TCM believes that the best cure is prevention.

No other healing system is built on a complete philosophical and theoretical specialty in prevention. My mission is to let people know the critical role prevention plays in saving our lives. Minor conditions that many Westerners would shrug off cause the TCM patient to run to her doctor. A well-educated TCM patient knows that addressing these health issues today can help her stay healthier and live longer tomorrow. This principle is particularly true when it comes to women's problems. Sometimes, I feel so sorry for women in Western society. I believe that women have been conditioned to view and accept their menstrual irregularities, PMS, migraine headaches, bloating, and constipation, among a host of other symptoms, as the price of being female. From the information on the breast cancer progression chart in Chapter 3, we've seen that nothing could be farther from the truth. Unfortunately, women don't know that these frequent symptoms can actually be eliminated with acupuncture and herbs. If your body is healthy, this kind of monthly suffering does not occur. According to TCM, it is not normal to have problems with your menstrual cycle. I always tell my patients that any problems with the menstrual cycle means that they already have a liver dysfunction.

Let's revisit our car analogy. TCM understands the conditions mentioned above as serious internal signals from the body that it's beginning to "run on empty." These signals are red flags that its organs, meridians, or overall Qi have become unbalanced. Left uncorrected, these conditions eventually can lead to something as serious as breast cancer. One of the most important parts of my mission is to help all women understand the root cause of breast cancer. When you understand this, then you will be more sensitive and respond to early warning signals that should be taken seriously. Some of these serious signals are outlined in Chapter 8.

How did TCM come to this deeper understanding of breast cancer? More than five hundred years ago, TCM had already identified the root cause of breast cancer. It also understood how to prevent it, or—once contracted—how to control it. This knowledge, along with related treatments based on TCM principles, has been passed down from generation to generation and, as we have seen, is still used today in China to treat breast cancer successfully. This knowledge is also used side-by-side with Western-style treatments in certain Chinese hospitals to enhance breast cancer treatment. It is applied in scores of universities dedicated to teaching TCM exclusively and training TCM practitioners.

❧TCM views and treats the human body as an organic whole

TCM, above all, sees the human body as an organic whole, a complete system made up of physical structures, emotions, mind, and spirit. It does not separate your body into parts, nor does it treat just one part of your body. In the TCM view, everything in the body is seen as woven together into a seamless whole; all parts have a relationship with one another. And, TCM relies on an ancient framework, the Five Element Theory, to help guide its understanding. The human body is made up of viscera, bowels, tissues, and other physical structures. Each has its own physiological function; all of them together comprise the web of life of an individual. It is important to note that TCM believes that emotional, mental, and spiritual capacities are as important as the body's physical properties in terms of health. For example, the emotion connected with the liver is anger. Anger is a normal human emotion. If you experience it and let it go, you can remain healthy. But, if you suffer from chronic anger or constantly hold anger deep within you in some way, you can eventually disrupt the normal healthy functioning of your liver. What does this mean?

One of the liver's main jobs is to promote the smooth flow of Qi and blood throughout the body. It is also responsible for the smooth flow of emotions. If it starts sputtering and performing its job poorly or unevenly, this condition can then cause menstrual cycle disorders such as PMS, cramps, and headaches. Chronic anger can also be the true source of breast tenderness, uterine fibroids, and stomach distention. You may not notice it, but when your life is going smoothly, your periods are regular and other female problems are less intense.

❧TCM understands that the human body has an inseparable connection with the natural world and the Universe

Although we may not be conscious of it and our lifestyles may prevent us from sensing it, each of us lives within nature and is subject to natural laws. Whether we want to accept it or not, we are affected directly and indirectly by changes in nature, geographical locations, alternations of the earth and earth energies, the movement of the seasons, the movement of the sun and moon, and the time of day, among other things. These deep connections were well understood by practitioners of TCM thousands of years ago; today, they are reflected in the recent scientific work on biorhythms, quantum physics, and bioelectromagnetics.

As early as 219 A.D., the *Shang Han Lun,* a book written by Zhang Zhongjing, discussed the particular times of day when herbal medicines would have the best effect on the patient. This principle is perhaps best captured by the TCM treatment protocol that diagnosis, treatment, and prevention always depend on: "Who you are, where you are, when you are, and how you are." This means that all the following factors must play a role in effective diagnosis and treatment: geographical location, season, time of day, genetics, and age, as well as the condition of the body. With so many factors, you can begin to appreciate the complexity of a medicine that believes no two people are exactly alike. All of TCM is focused on treating the individual—as an individual. How does it go about this? It works first to bring your body into harmony within itself, and then to help it come into harmony with the Universe in which it lives.

Here's one famous ancient story called "The Yellow Jar." It shows how important your energy connection with your own location is. Long ago, TCM recognized what many of today's global travelers experience—location sickness. That is, they understood that for many reasons, a foreign environment can have a negative health affect.

In the distant past, in the ancient Chinese province of Wei, there lived a merchant named Wang. His stock-in-trade were richly colored brocaded silks. A very prosperous man, Wang spent most of the year traveling north and south, east and west, supplying all parts of the country with his beautiful wares.

On one such trip, a local village supplier asked of Wang, "How do you manage? If I traveled one half the time and distance as you, I would be homesick all the time." "Well, since you've been a good and loyal customer all these years, I'll tell you the secret of my success," Wang replied. Then, he opened his coat and pulled forth a small yellow ceramic jar. "This," Wang said lovingly holding the jar, "is dirt from my beloved native Wei. When the road has been my home for many months, all I do is make a simple porridge and add a pinch of earth. All my homesickness vanishes. I feel restored!"

What this wise merchant understood is that while Universal energy remains constant, the energy of the earth varies. Each village, state, and country has its own special energy essence. It is this particular "Qi of place" that is acutely missed both by the body and the emotions when homesickness or physical illness takes hold. Traditionally, earth or uncooked rice from the home village was carried while traveling or upon a move to a different region. A small amount mixed into food or drink would transfer the essence of "home."

I like to remind my patients and students that in this age of nonstop global travel, it's good to remember that we are rooted to the Qi or energy of a specific place and can still connect with it through simple actions like this. I use this principle to tell my patients who travel to bring some food from home. Even small packages of oatmeal can help them stay balanced and healthy, as well as avoid jet lag while they go through changes in time and place.

I find these stories very interesting because they illustrate so well how certain intangible things can affect our physical bodies. This individualized approach allows TCM to make an informed diagnosis only when it takes into account the specifics of "who you are," "where you are," "when you are," and "how you are." It opens a window for TCM to see deeply into the root cause of health problems and go to their source. While its specialty is prevention, TCM does not suppress or cover up symptoms when they're encountered.

APPLYING TCM PRINCIPLES
TO BREAST CANCER

Let's look at how these principles bear on breast cancer. According to TCM, the root cause of breast cancer is a two-part condition: it involves the stagnation of Qi in the meridians that run through the breast area, and the dysfunction of one or more of three major organs—kidney, stomach, and liver. (When TCM discusses an organ, its meaning is broader than the physical organ. It includes its energy function as well.) This stagnation and dysfunction are mainly caused by excessive emotional energy that has built up over time and manifested itself physically.

Following are several descriptions of the root cause of breast cancer outlined in ancient medical texts.

❧ "When liver energy stagnates, it can cause the lower energy gate to close. When this gates closes, energy cannot run smoothly through the lower part of the body which can cause menstrual disorders. This condition can lead to breast cancer."

Dr. Zhen-Heng Zhu (circa 1300 A.D.)

❧ "These [negative] emotions accumulate day by day and cause spleen and stomach Qi deficiency and liver Qi stagnation. These conditions will cause the body to create a lump. When Qi stagnates in the meridians over time, a small seed can progress to a cancerous mass. Then the five major organs will spiral out of balance. The problem is called breast cancer."

Dr. Chen, *Wai Ke Zheng Zong* (circa 1400 A.D.)

❧ "Breast cancer is caused by the damaged Qi of the liver and spleen/stomach. Also, the Qi of both the liver and stomach has stagnated."

Dr. Qian Wu, Qing Dynasty (circa 1600 A.D.)

TCM theory states that as long as the body's two major operating systems work in harmony both within themselves and with each other, good health will be maintained and disease avoided. It is as simple and, as we shall see, as complex as that! Let's look at these two critical systems that also encompass the Western concept of the immune system.

   ❧ The meridian network or web of energy pathways: TCM states that even if you have a genetic or hereditary predisposition to breast cancer, as long as Qi, or vital energy, flows smoothly through the body's meridians in the breast area, you can reduce your risk of breast cancer. You can think of the meridian network as a highway system—there are superhighways, two-lane highways, local streets, and small alleys. If a blockage occurs at one of the major intersections, a traffic jam will follow. In much the same way, if an energy blockage occurs in your body, your Qi will begin to block up in a particular meridian. If unrelieved, the blocked Qi can eventually produce a physical mass. This mass, in turn, depending on other factors, can take a quantum leap and turn into breast cancer. Interestingly, scientists are beginning to duplicate this ancient theory in laboratories where the manipulation of energy flows can be made to produce matter.

   ❧ The five major organs: TCM states as long as the five major organs (kidney, spleen, liver, heart, and lung) and their respective companion organs (bladder, stomach, gallbladder, small intestine, large intestine) function in harmony together, even with a genetic or hereditary predisposition to breast cancer, your body has the necessary strength to control cancer's energy pattern and prevent it from developing. And even if breast cancer develops, you have a much better chance of healing if you are working toward this state where the organs work in harmony and Qi flows in the meridians. You will learn a lot more about these organs in Chapter 7.

The healthy functioning of these two major operating systems has special importance for women predisposed to breast cancer. Why? Because if we shift our thinking a bit and adopt the TCM point of view, we can see how breast cancer begins and develops when the proper internal environment occurs. For example, why doesn't breast cancer develop in women predisposed to it when they are age ten, or fifteen, or even at twenty-five? Why did their inherited and genetic traits like hair and blood types, eye shape, etc., appear immediately at the moment of birth? Why do some mothers get breast cancer at age fifty and survive, while their daughters get the same disease at forty and die? In each case, the answer lies within the individual and how healthy her two major operating systems. This is where the power to control the genetic seed resides.

THE TCM DEFINITION OF CANCER: QI DEFICIENCY, COLD, AND STAGNATION

Ancient practitioners recognized that when there is cancer, three major conditions are present: Qi deficiency, cold, and stagnation. Cancer carries a cold or yin energy. Its very essence is cold or frozen. That's why heat treatments with lasers and infrared lights are currently being explored to eliminate cancerous growths. Qi deficiency (which means your organs do not have enough Qi to perform their natural functions) can lead to cold. If a Qi deficiency continues over time, it will inevitably cause Qi or blood stagnation (which means that these intertwined forces become blocked in their natural, healthy flow through the body). When this condition occurs, a lump or mass will inevitably develop. The condition of stagnation then means the body's internal environment will become cold. If the body is further insulted by external cold, this condition will worsen. If you have cancer, no matter what kind, these three conditions will always be present: Qi deficiency, blood stagnation, and cold in the meridians or specific organs. I urge you to take good care of yourself if you suffer from one or more of these conditions. Your body now offers the right environment for cancer to develop. To prevent or treat breast cancer, TCM has many treatments to address these particular conditions. The first thing practitioners do is try to increase overall Qi, then break up any stagnation, and then relieve cold.

HOW EMOTIONS CONTRIBUTE TO THE ROOT CAUSE OF BREAST CANCER

The *Nei Jing* states "All disease comes from Qi stagnation." In this case, the ancient medical text refers to emotional Qi. Let's look at the seven emotions or seven different kinds of emotional reactions that can directly or indirectly cause Qi stagnation. These are emotions you have in response to events that happen in your life. Each emotion is connected to a specific organ (You can see them in the Five Element Theory chart on page 84.) These emotions are: joy, anger, sadness or melancholy, anxiety, grief, fear, and terror. For most people, these emotions usually remain within a normal range. If sudden, violent or chronic emotional stimuli affect your body beyond its ability to adapt or endure them, they will actually cause a functional disorder of a specific organ and its Qi. These emotional stimuli can then become pathogenic (disease or illness-causing) factors. Because TCM treats the whole person, it has always recognized emotions as causative factors in health problems. Its classical texts refer to this condition as "internal injury by seven emotions." In the case of breast cancer, we shall see how anger, the emotion of the liver, plays a central role.

Let's look more closely at several of these emotions that can cause an organ function disorder or stagnation of Qi or blood in the meridians. They usually affect the organ when there is an excess of the emotion, but a deficiency can also have a negative impact. It is important to understand that the five organ pairs and their emotions share a reciprocal relationship. That means anger can damage your liver, and it is possible that a liver condition can generate an emotional imbalance. Remember TCM sees your body's ideal healthy state as having balance and harmony in all things:

❧ Joy and happiness are related to the heart. Believe it or not, you can actually be too happy. If you experience an excess of happiness, you will cause your blood to become out of control. This condition can, in turn, cause a mental problem or even a heart attack. This really happens, not just in the movies!

❧ Anger is related to the liver. If you're always angry, or you have difficulty letting negative emotions go, you will cause liver Qi stagnation. This stagnation can lead to headaches, stomach problems, tendon problems, and more. TCM considers the liver the major organ for women's health. If you're under a lot of stress, you will eventually develop a liver function disorder, you might develop migraine headaches, constant stomachaches, or brittle nails. Almost certainly, you will experience menstrual cycle problems. TCM also relates infertility to liver function disorder or liver Qi stagnation.

❧ Worry is related to the spleen. If you always worry or continually over-think, you will cause stomach and spleen Qi stagnation. In this case, you might lose your appetite, have digestive system problems, retain water, find it difficult to lose weight and, for women, bruise easily. Women on diets can become increasingly frustrated with their efforts to lose weight if they don't understand that worry or over-thinking effectively stops the function of the spleen/stomach organ pair.

Here's a case study that illustrates this point. I once had a patient who worried about almost everything. She was actually too thin, but she wanted to join my weight management class to try and understand the source of her problem better. When she began, she complained that she never wanted to eat anything. Her appetite was virtually gone. During class, I wanted to help her, so I created a situation that would make her liver Qi rise. I started a discussion which I knew would make her angry. (I also knew this would activate her liver Qi.) That day she became so angry that she stomped out. I explained to the class what happened and why. I told them that I was not angry with her, but that I was using ancient Chinese psychology. In this case, I knew her excess anger would cause her liver Qi to rise. This, in turn, would reconnect with the stomach's Qi and thereby restart the stomach's function and help her appetite return. We spoke about this and the next week she came back to tell the class that after the angry exchange, her appetite underwent a tremendous change. She found that she could eat normally again and reported that for the first time in a long time she was feeling much better.

❦ Sadness belongs to the lung. If you're always sad, or you experience sudden deep sadness, you will cause a lung Qi deficiency and lung Qi stagnation. When this occurs, you can develop a cough, experience chest tightness, and skin problems (the skin is the "tissue" of the lung). You will also experience digestive system problems like constipation (the lung shares an energy relationship with the large intestine).

❦ Fear and terror are the emotions that can affect the kidney. Fear is an internal condition, while terror comes from outside factors. Both can cause a kidney Qi disorder. If you continually feel fear or are suddenly confronted with a situation that strikes terror into your heart (real or imagined), you might experience cold in the body, or lower back pain. You might lose your hair, suddenly or gradually, or your ears (the "opening" of the kidney) may ring. You may experience frequent urination and even develop osteoporosis (bones are the "excess" of the kidney).

In "Plain Questions," a part of the ancient medical text known as the *Nei Jing,* it says: "Rage causes adverse upward flow of the liver-Qi, excessive joy relaxes the heart-Qi, excessive sorrow leads to the consumption of Qi, fear causes the sinking of kidney-Qi . . . fright interrupts the flow of Qi, anxiety causes the stagnation of spleen-Qi." Remember that these emotions have a reciprocal relationship with their corresponding organs. A problem with the liver can cause anger; conversely anger can cause a liver disorder. The same kind of correspondences holds true for the other emotions.

These seven emotions can not only cause illness, but also aggravate it. For instance, the course of many health problems is affected by the ups and downs of the patient's moods or emotions. TCM pays particular attention to the mental state of the patient and her need for consolation and comfort through an illness to help influence a positive outcome. The best doctor not only treats the problem, but recognizes that the whole person is struggling with it. He or she does as much as possible to offer as much emotional and psychological support as possible. In the thirteenth century, hundreds of years before Sigmund Freud, the father of Western psychoanalysis, Chinese doctors were already using well-developed psychological theories based on their understanding of the dynamics of emotions. You might find the following examples very interesting. There are several others in Chapter 9.

ANGER CAUSES ACNE

An elementary school teacher in her early thirties came to see if I could do anything to relieve an acute acne condition that had developed rather suddenly. After performing a TCM diagnosis, we sat down to talk. It turned out that she was quite stressed. Not only was her job caring for a classroom full of third grade children difficult, but something traumatic had recently happened to her.

This woman was very sad because she and her boyfriend of several years had planned to marry in the near future. Her boyfriend, however, had just met someone else and within a few weeks of seeing this woman had told my patient that he was planning to marry the new woman. Needless to say this devastated my patient.

Her sadness was only surpassed by her anger, which was with her constantly. It was anger that she tried to hide, but it kept on boiling deep within her. After several weeks, she developed severe acne all over her face. She also developed stomach cramps and severe constipation. These physical conditions only added to her pain and suffering.

As we talked, I encouraged my patient to explore different ways to look at what had happened to her. I told her that everyone has a right to love the person they think they love. Because her boyfriend chose to marry a woman he barely knew, it meant that this woman's attraction was far stronger than hers. I told her she should consider herself lucky because this meeting might have taken place after she had married her boyfriend. The result would have been the same; he would have left and she would have been devastated, perhaps even more so.

I urged her to let her deep anger and sadness go. To help her, I gave her a classical TCM herbal formula that works to unblock liver Qi and promote its smooth flow throughout the body. After taking the herbs for two weeks, her acne began to disappear; then her stomach pain went away, and finally the constipation stopped.

This woman was very interested in her treatment and how to get better. I explained that because she held her anger so deeply inside and this event had affected her so violently, her liver Qi had become stuck. (The liver and its Qi are responsible for the smooth flow of blood, Qi and emotions.) When this happens, the whole body's Qi becomes stuck or stagnates. Then the body must find a way to relieve itself; it struggles to rebalance its Qi, otherwise it will become even sicker. In my patient's case, two conditions helped me understand clearly the root cause of her problems: stomach cramps and constipation. Both the stomach and large intestine meridians run through the face. In this particular person, her body handled liver Qi stagnation by trying to relieve itself through the acne and acute stomach problems.

Because the root cause of her physical problems was connected to the underlying emotional problem of anger, the TCM herbs could only take her so far by addressing the symptoms. I told her that to truly heal, she had to help herself by learning to let her anger go, then this kind of acne would never bother her again. Her stomach pain and constipation would also go away.

It's important to understand that the very real phenomenon of blocked or stagnated Qi was the catalyst for the physical problems that developed. Because of the nature and location of the physical problems, they were readily traceable by TCM diagnosis to their root cause. This woman's unhappy event had unbalanced the healthy connections between her body, emotions, and spirit.

HOW DIET AND LIFESTYLE CONTRIBUTE TO THE ROOT CAUSE OF BREAST CANCER

TCM says that the kidney is the foundation of your health before you are born. This Qi is what sustains you in the womb. After birth, the spleen and stomach become the foundation of good health. Also, their partnership with the liver is essential.

That is why your daily diet plays the central role in warding off illness or disease. Your everyday routine affects your health more than any single thing you can name. TCM believes that improper diet, too much work, and not enough rest will affect the physiological functions of your organs and reduce your resistance to diseases. It thus considers that these important lifestyle choices can become pathogenic, or disease-producing, factors.

Let's go into this more deeply. As with all things, moderation is the key, especially when it comes to eating. Excessive hunger or excessive eating can both give rise to illness. In the former, taking in too little food can result in too little material available to be transformed into Qi and blood. This situation eventually leads to the deficiency or weakness of both of these vital elements and brings on illness. Another effect is that it can seriously compromise the body's ability to resist external pathogens, like colds and viruses, etc. Overeating beyond the normal ability of one's digestion can also bring on a host of problems, including (no surprise) common indigestion. Sometimes, it can lead to more serious conditions like food retention, acid reflux, vomiting, diarrhea, and other conditions. TCM texts say: "Excessive diet impairs the intestines and stomach." Not eating regularly and at normal intervals can cause a stomach function disorder. Unhygienic diets can also lead to various kinds of gastrointestinal diseases like food poisoning and parasitoses.

Food preferences also influence health. TCM says that a proper, balanced mixture of high-quality foods provides good nourishment. Any excessive food preference may cause a disharmony of yin and yang energies, nutritional deficiency and illness. This is particularly relevant to breast cancer prevention. A continual preference for cold or uncooked foods and foods with a cold essence can affect the stomach and its meridian.

This key meridian runs up through the breast area; this area is where 50 percent of all breast cancers are diagnosed. A preference for dry hot food can cause stomach heat; a rich fatty diet can cause carbuncles. Many women have the experience of craving a specific taste, especially during their periods. Addiction or craving of one of the five flavors (sour, bitter, sweet, acid, and salty) can also create illness. You can tell which organ is out of balance by the taste or flavor you crave. The five flavors are listed below.

Organ	Liver	Heart	Spleen	Lung	Kidney
Taste	Sour	Bitter	Sweet	Acid	Salty

I constantly talk with my Western women patients about their eating habits. I remind them that without a good digestive system, they cannot get enough energy support to fight breast cancer. This is very important for women undergoing chemotherapy or radiation, which has already damaged their digestive system. I also have a great many patients who tell me proudly the amount of vitamins, nutritional supplements, nutraceuticals, tonics, etc., they take. I know they think they are doing the right thing, but I must tell them that without a well-functioning digestive system, their body simply cannot absorb what goes into it. I tell them: "Look at it this way, if you have a food grinder and several of the blades are dull and the whole machine can't draw enough power to operate at the proper speed, do you think it will efficiently process everything you throw into it?" TCM believes your body has the innate capability of extracting Qi to power it from a balanced diet to keep you healthy. In other words, a calcium deficiency cannot be treated by calcium supplements alone. Why? TCM states that the bones are the "tissue" of the kidney. Weak bones point to weak kidney function. The root cause of the calcium deficiency is kidney Qi deficiency. Without treating the kidney, you cannot treat the true origin of this problem.

A reasonable workload and sufficient rest are also essential to good health. This is simple to say, but almost impossible to do, with our stressed-out lifestyles. Any time your body is overstrained, which can encompass physical, mental or sexual overexertion, you put yourself at risk for disease. Each of these states affects the body's Qi and creates the root cause of many health problems. For instance, physical overexertion can cause Qi exhaustion. Mild cases show up as fatigue, mental or physical; severe cases manifest themselves as tendon injuries, muscle or bone problems, arthralgia, myalgia of the limbs, among other conditions. Mental overstrain will cause insomnia, abdominal distention, loose stool, and more. Excessive sexual activity, because it impairs the function of the kidney, can lead to tinnitus, listlessness, impotence, and more. In the pursuit of creating balance and harmony in all things, there can also be such a thing as overrest. No motion, no daily activity, or a total lack of exercise, can impede the free flow of Qi. This can manifest itself as listlessness, loss of appetite, shortness of breath on exertion, palpitation or obesity. Too much rest can actually impair the body's resistance to diseases and make it weak and susceptible to an attack from external pathogens.

HOW YOUR GENETIC MAKEUP CONTRIBUTES TO THE ROOT CAUSE OF BREAST CANCER

Chinese medicine is always concerned with a patient's genetic information. This information is directly related to the kidney's Qi and its function. For example, if you have had a premature birth, you did not receive enough kidney support from the combined Qi of your parents. This means that some kind of problem may hide in your body and show up later in life, as your inherited kidney Qi declines. To treat these kinds of things, Chinese medicine has used a special tea for centuries to help increase a pregnant woman's Qi, or vital energy. Beyond that, it has an entire philosophy of treating the pregnant woman through a special diet and emotional and lifestyle prescriptions to prevent problems in the unborn child. What if you're born with a genetic problem? Even with this kind of seed, for a genetic problem to develop, your body's defense systems must malfunction. Today, for those women who are at risk for breast cancer or whose close relatives have developed breast cancer, it is important to understand that, according to TCM theory, a genetic condition only can emerge if your own immune system loses its strength.

Let's see how this works. We asked this question earlier. If a mother gets breast cancer at age fifty and survives, then why does her daughter get breast cancer at age forty and not survive? The answer is that the daughter's body became so far out of balance much earlier than her mother's that her cancer's energy was able to totally take control. Her mother, on the other hand, had enough healing ability left in her body to control the cancer until she was a decade older. Again, I want to emphasize that the answer lies within the individual. What about a mother and sister who both have breast cancer, but their daughters do not? Often these younger women with the genetic marker for cancer face the agonizing decision of having a mastectomy without having cancer. Is this really a lifesaving operation? According to TCM, you may be cutting off the branch, but you have not uprooted the entire tree. In other words, the genetic seed, the DNA time bomb, is still somewhere within the body. If the right conditions occur, which we've mentioned above, you still are at serious risk for cancer.

Chinese medicine sees genetic problems as internal seeds, which require certain conditions to flourish. Once the seed and requirements meet, there is nothing that can stop the process of growth. It's like the flowers in your garden. When you plant them and provide the right temperature and the right amount of moisture, you can pretty well be assured that they will grow. They keep growing until they reach the end of their natural lifespan of lifecycle, or you cut them down. If these requirements aren't present, your seed will never grow. While you might inherit a cancer seed from your parents, if your body doesn't provide the right conditions for growth, how will it develop?

HOW SIX EXTERNAL CLIMATE CONDITIONS CONTRIBUTE TO THE ROOT CAUSE OF BREAST CANCER

TCM defines six climatic conditions that, in excess, it considers pathogenic, or disease-causing. They are: wind, the heat of summer, fire, dampness, dryness, and cold. Because they are normal climatic conditions of nature, they are also referred to as "six natural factors." Because human beings are fairly adaptable, they can live in a wide variety of climates without too much trouble. The six natural factors can not actually cause people to develop illness or contract disease. But, if a person's Qi is weak or unable to adapt to climate changes, these factors can affect them negatively. This is particularly true if these changes are excessive, or insufficient, or unseasonable, or if they occur too quickly and too violently. I think many of you can relate to severe headaches that come along as the barometer drops. I help quite a number of patients with arthritis pain. Different kinds of arthritis respond to different weather patterns. Some people tell me that they are much better at predicting the weather than our local weatherman. Interestingly, many of these people have old sports injuries that were treated many years ago with ice to help relieve pain and swelling.

I tell my arthritis patients that inside their body, they have conditions of wind and cold. When the outside conditions match, their body automatically responds to this energy change. Some people find the cold intolerable; I suggest they go to warmer climates, if possible. Those who are affected by dampness do much better in dryer climates.

When they begin to affect the body, TCM refers to the six natural factors as six yin (excess), or six exogenous, factors.

We know that sometimes spring sees more problems due to wind; summer brings on heat problems; fall creates dryness; winter, cold. If you live in damp conditions for a long time, you can eventually be affected by dampness. The same is true of living in places that regularly record high temperatures. These yin factors can attack the body singly or together. The common cold and arthritis or arthralgia are two examples.

Most people don't realize it, but these factors can cause diseases by entering the body through the skin or the mouth or through both of them. The foreign invaders that enter can be bacterial, viral, physical, chemical, among others.

Wind

What can wind do? Wind that is pathogenic can occur in all seasons. The *Nei Jing* states that wind is the beginning of all illness. Pathogenic wind tends to rise and move up and outward; it has the ability to penetrate the skin barrier. This kind of wind usually affects the upper body, skin and muscles, and frequently causes headaches, dizziness, eye and mouth problems. Should the wind then migrate or travel within the body, it can end up causing pain in the joints or limbs. Diseases or illness caused by wind that migrates are very unpredictable. For example, a skin problem might show up suddenly in one place, then regress and reappear in another location. Tremors, convulsions, vertigo, and other problems of involuntary or vibrational movement are attributed by TCM to pathogenic wind. Other pathogenic factors actually attach themselves to wind and ride its energy into the human body. There they can create major problems that are often difficult and stubborn to treat.

Heat

TCM believes that summer heat is transformed from heat and fire. It comes from external factors. This pathogen is very hot in nature and it's derived from summer's scorching heat. When it attacks, the body responds with physical conditions like a high fever, a state of upset, a flushed face and a rapid pulse. Summer heat usually rises and disperses. It can consume Qi quickly and affect the body's delicate balance of fluids. This kind of heat, which is different from fire, causes many symptoms like excess thirst, dry lips and tongue, light flow of urine with a dark color. You probably have seen the effects of summer heat many times—especially at the beach. It can cause profuse perspiration. If that happens, naturally, Qi is also lost because it is intertwined with perspiration's fluid. A Qi deficiency can then cause shortness of breath, lassitude, and abrupt fainting and even loss of consciousness. Often, we see summer heat with another natural factor—dampness.

Fire

Fire has the same nature as warmth and heat, it is just more intense. Often patients hear their TCM practitioner describe certain conditions as being related to fire. The fire they are describing may come from outside factors, for instance foods that are barbecued or deep-fried foods. The second kind of fire is when internal energy has accumulated and gone beyond the smoldering stagnation stage to the further degree of internal fire. The ancient Chinese characterized fire as the "excess of Qi." Other pathogens can transform themselves into fire and cause conditions that are related to the qualities of fire. For example, fire tends to burn and scorch. Its disease often appears in such symptoms as high fever, flushed face, blood-shot eyes, dislike of heat, constipation, a red tongue with a yellow coating. Fire also tends to rise upwards and its symptoms usually manifest themselves in the upper body, especially the face and head. Heart-fire can appear as a reddened tongue-tip; stomach-fire can flare up and cause swollen gums; liver-fire can show up in swollen, congested eyes. Fire also tends to burn up body fluid and Qi. When this kind of pathogenic fire attacks, it will force body fluid to leak out. This will impair yin fluids and cause conditions of thirst, dryness in the throat and mouth, scanty urine, and constipation.

If you have fire in your liver, you will see it manifest in very red or bloodshot eyes. In some cases pathogenic fire can accelerate blood flow so much that various bleeding symptoms occur. When fire enters the blood system carbuncles and sores can develop. If the fire rises, you may experience sores in your mouth or on your face. If the fire descends, then you may develop vaginal sores or even herpes. Fire also has the capability to irritate the heart, its corresponding organ, as well as the spirit. If you have fire in your heart, you might have nightmares; or the tip of your tongue may burn frequently. One of the heart's main jobs is to govern the vessels and house the *Shen* or spirit. In mild cases of pathogenic fire, there may be some upset or insomnia. In severe cases, conditions like mania, restlessness, delirium, mental illness, and even unconsciousness, can occur.

Dampness

Dampness usually occurs in late summer, just as it turns into autumn. The fall season, as many of us know, is when illnesses and diseases of dampness take hold. Again, TCM divides pathogenic dampness into two kinds: one is external and is due to the dampness of climate, being in water continually, or being caught in the rain. The other is an internal kind of dampness. Internal dampness results when the spleen suffers from a dysfunction and cannot perform one of its very important jobs—transporting fluids and managing water metabolism. I often tell my patients that they should avoid overeating raw vegetables, or drinking too many cold things. Believe it or not, this kind of diet with its excess cold and dampness, will unbalance the healthy function of the stomach. The stomach's main love is all things warm. If you have a white, thick coating on your tongue, you already have internal dampness.

Characteristics of the first kind of dampness are that it is heavy and turbid in nature. Individuals complain of heavy feelings, lassitude, heavy sensations of the head and body. Sometimes they will describe aching limbs that are heavy and slow to move. Excess secretions can also indicate signs of dampness. These can include eye matter, loose stool, or stool with mucous, pus or blood, among others.

Health conditions of dampness usually follow a long course; they often linger and are stubborn to cure. The natural direction for dampness is downward. TCM states that symptoms of dampness are found primarily in the lower body. I advise women to be careful of dampness because it is considered a yin pathogen and can block or obstruct the movement of Qi. Faulty spleen function can also hold water in the body and cause weight retention and other weight problems, which are difficult to fix.

Dryness

TCM considers autumn a dry season when water is in short supply. This is when the condition of dryness rules. There are two type of pathogenic dryness. Diseases caused by the first kind are related to environmental factors. When it attacks, this pathogen usually makes its way in through the mouth and nose to the lung. It affects the defensive or *wei* Qi and the lung. It is easy to see this kind of disease-provoking agent in action in the fall. You can go to any park on a nice warm fall day and see people without their sweaters, or walking around in shorts.

They believe that the weather is still summer-like. It does feel that way, but this is not the same season or the same energy as summer. Consequently, these people often are among the first to pick up a cold or the flu. Their cold may be accompanied by a fever; they may have dryness in the mouth and nose, dryness in their throats, a dry cough, dryness of the skin, and sometimes constipation. To a TCM doctor, these kinds of symptoms coupled with the season offer a clue to the real source of the patient's condition.

Pathogenic dryness attacks the lung, an organ TCM considers very delicate. It is even called the "baby organ." Its natural preference is moisture and it dislikes dryness. The lung's "tissues" are the skin and hair of the body surfaces. Its opening is the nose. If you have dry skin that doesn't respond to any kind of cream or topical treatment, you most likely have a condition of internal dryness of the lung. Chemotherapy and radiation can have a tremendous effect on lung function. Look up specific foods like pears and kiwi whose essence can relieve excess lung heat and recipes to help treat this condition in Chapter 17.

Cold

Cold is an aspect of all seasons, not just winter. Many patients have heard their TCM practitioner diagnose their condition as one of cold. TCM categorizes two types of pathogenic cold: one is environmental in nature; the other is a state where the individual's yang-Qi is deficient. With the second type, the internal energies of yin and yang have tipped out of balance. The body can no longer maintain a normal level of warmth. Those suffering from pathogenic cold usually have an aversion to cold. If it attacks the spleen and stomach, the individual may experience abdominal pain that is cold in nature. How do you know your stomach pain comes from cold? If your condition responds to treatments of warmth, like heating pads, hot water bottles, the warmth of your hand, or drinking hot fluids with herbs that have a warm essence, like ginger or cinnamon, then your pain comes from pathogenic cold. Often, women with PMS or menstrual cramps have conditions of internal cold. I strongly recommend that they avoid drinking ice cold drinks or eating cold foods during this time. This kind of cold is one that coagulates and obstructs things that it encounters. Within the body, cold has the power to block or stagnate Qi, as well as blood, in the meridians and interfere with their flow. This, in turn, can cause all kinds of pain. You can see how serious cold is by rereading TCM's definition of the three conditions that are present with cancer: Qi deficiency, cold, and stagnation.

Another effect that cold has on the body is constriction. Pathogenic cold has the ability to constrict the function of Qi in various organs. This means it can cause the body's physical structures like muscles, tendons, etc., to contract and, in some cases, go into a spasm. Let's look at what happens when pathogenic cold attacks. One thing it can do is cause the sweat pores and muscle structures to contract or close. The defensive yang-qi can stagnate and not flow upward. This state can cause an aversion to cold and bring on a fever, which is called anhidrosis (or lack of sweating). Or, it can cause cramps and make joint extension difficult.

Organ	Liver	Heart	Spleen	Lung	Kidney
Climate	Wind	Fire Summer Heat	Dampness	Dryness Summer Heat	Cold

Each of these climate factors alone, or in combination, can adversely affect the body and unbalance the workings of Qi, the meridians, or the five organs. These are the conditions that open the door to the root cause of breast cancer.

HOW ENVIRONMENTAL FACTORS CONTRIBUTE TO THE ROOT CAUSE OF BREAST CANCER

Environmental factors can very easily contribute to the root cause of breast cancer. As we've seen, your body runs on Qi or energy. It is entirely possible that a wide range of environmental factors can interfere with the healthy functioning of the body. For instance, strong electrical fields can interfere with or change your body's own electrical field. New scientific work with bio-electromagnetics at Stanford University in California shows that even very subtle frequencies far below what was originally considered "safe" can create cellular changes. Electrical fields have the ability to disrupt the energy flow of your meridians. In addition, they can "sap" your energy and cause a serious Qi deficiency. The stronger the field, the worse the effect. From my experience, I often find that patients who constantly work with computers or in laboratories with microwaves have neck and shoulder pain that is very difficult to treat and take much longer than others to see some benefit.

Be especially careful if you work around radiation. Your immune system could become weakened by this kind of energy force. If you are continually exposed to these kinds of energies, you are at risk for compromising your own self-healing ability.

We also know that certain kinds of chemicals can either directly or indirectly cause cancer. Even if you don't directly touch a toxic chemical, simply smelling it can interrupt the smooth and healthy functioning of your lung. Why? According to TCM theory, the sense organ associated with the lung is the nose. Smelling toxic substances allows their energy to penetrate straight to the nose's related organ, the lung, which is responsible for controlling the distribution of Qi throughout your body. Tampering with the lung can bring on extreme fatigue, and other conditions of serious exhaustion. The lung also controls the health of the skin. If your lung function is disrupted, then your skin can be affected. This also provides some insight into just how damaging smoking can be.

You spend the largest part of your day at your job. You invest a lot of emotional, physical, mental, and spiritual energy in your work environment. If you don't like your job, but you must keep it, then your mind and spirit are in conflict and under constant pressure. This condition can cause internal energy stagnation in any organ or meridian. If you always find yourself in this situation, physical problems will eventually show up somewhere in your body. For instance, during your menstrual cycle, you may experience PMS, headaches, sleep problems, breast tenderness, and so on. You may not relate these symptoms to your chronic emotional distress, but according to TCM theories, this is the root cause of the physical discomfort.

Stress takes a deadly toll on the liver, which is the most important organ for women's health. If the function of your liver is out of balance, then you might experience physical discomfort in the form of symptoms such as menstrual disorders, PMS, stomach distention or bloating, nail problems, and itchy and/or red eyes. If the liver continues to be stressed over time, this condition can lead to function disorders of other critical organs, such as the stomach, kidney, heart, and lung.

It is vital to find a healthy way to deal with the stress in your life. Try not to absorb the negative energy of stress into your own energy system, but find productive ways to let it go. Acupuncture, yoga, and meditation, as well as certain Chinese herbal formulas, can help relieve stress. The *Wu Ming* Meridian Therapy movements in the Breast Cancer Prevention Project can also help reduce the chronic stress in your life. They work by helping you unite your body, mind, and spirit.

Many people exist in a hectic working environment. When lunch time comes, women often find themselves working and eating at the same time. This is not a healthy habit. Each activity needs its own energy source. If you do both at the same time, then your digestive system does not get sufficient energy to do its job. You may not be able to gain maximum nutrition from the food you're eating while you're working. If you always do this, then you can literally unbalance the normal functioning of your stomach, and you may experience stomachaches after eating. Because 50 percent of breast cancers appear in the area through which the stomach meridians run, it is critical to keep this organ and its meridians functioning well. Once you understand this, you can see why a simple thing like taking twenty minutes out of your day to eat your lunch in an unhurried manner can help you remain healthy.

While you don't have to love the people you work with, it's very important to have a harmonious work environment. Otherwise, your body will spend extra Qi to deal with emotional issues on a daily basis. This emotional discomfort can cause a function disorder of one or more organs. According to TCM theories, the root cause of breast cancer is closely related to holding unbalanced and/or excess emotions in the body. Held over time, this negative energy can stagnate and cause serious damage. It is not the experience of the emotion that is damaging—this is only being human. It is the holding of the excess emotion that causes problems. It is important to find healthy ways to release these emotions and become good at "letting things go."

Again, because you spend so many of your waking hours in the workplace, it is necessary to create harmony in your environment to the best of your ability. This way your body does not have to use up extra Qi just to maintain its normal function. Even a few small changes can help. When a plant flowers, it is at the peak of its energy. Try to bring a fresh flower into your workspace often to experience this special energy. This kind of "live" message can help your body recall its own healing energy. Place an evergreen plant near your computer. When your eyes become tired, change your field of vision to the plant. This can help you relieve eyestrain and help keep your vision healthy. Almost everyone can take a few short breaks during the workday. When you do, close your eyes and breathe slowly and deeply. Let everything go; do not focus on any problems or physical sensations or emotions. Many short meditations during the course of the day give the body a special energy recharge and can produce the same effect as a full twenty minutes of meditation. Getting into this habit can change your life and help you accumulate tremendous health benefits.

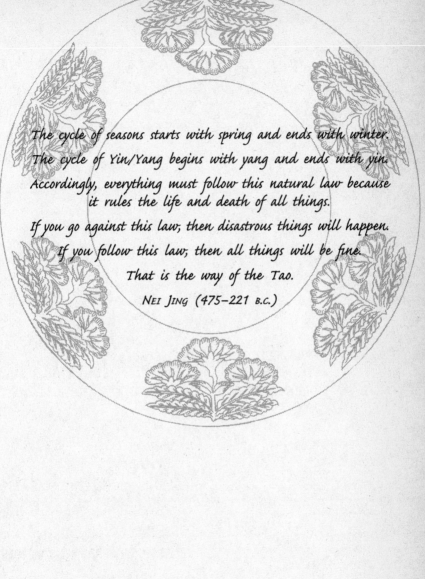

The cycle of seasons starts with spring and ends with winter.

The cycle of Yin/Yang begins with yang and ends with yin.

Accordingly, everything must follow this natural law because
it rules the life and death of all things.

If you go against this law, then disastrous things will happen.

If you follow this law, then all things will be fine.

That is the way of the Tao.

NEI JING (475–221 B.C.)

CHAPTER 6
Understanding the Basic Theories of TCM

As we have seen, the basic theories of TCM have been in place and unchanged for more than two thousand years. They are Yin and Yang, Qi and Blood, Five Element Theory, and Meridian Theory. The most important of these theories is Yin and Yang. This theory encompasses the eternal dance of the two complementary energies and constitutes the ultimate Universal law wherein all things must remain in harmony. As such, it is the foundation of all TCM, which seeks, above all, to keep the body in a condition of harmony both within itself and with the external world. As the *Nei Jing* says, "If you know the theory of Yin and Yang, you can be the best doctor . . . Without Yin/Yang, there is no life." Even the *Tao Te Ching*—a classical text written around the same time as the *Nei Jing*—says: "Yin and Yang are contained within all things." Qi is the intelligent force through which this theory manifests itself.

THE THEORY OF YIN AND YANG

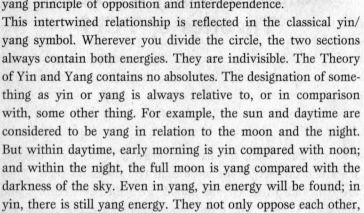

TCM believes everything is composed of two complementary energies: one energy is yin and the other is yang. They are never separate; one cannot exist without the other. This is the yin/yang principle of opposition and interdependence.

This intertwined relationship is reflected in the classical yin/yang symbol. Wherever you divide the circle, the two sections always contain both energies. They are indivisible. The Theory of Yin and Yang contains no absolutes. The designation of something as yin or yang is always relative to, or in comparison with, some other thing. For example, the sun and daytime are considered to be yang in relation to the moon and the night. But within daytime, early morning is yin compared with noon; and within the night, the full moon is yang compared with the darkness of the sky. Even in yang, yin energy will be found; in yin, there is still yang energy. They not only oppose each other, but are interdependent as well. You cannot have one without the other. This is Universal law at its simplest and deepest.

According to the Theory of Yin and Yang, male is yang; female is yin. Everything in the body is also under the control of yin and yang. For example, the front of the body is yin; the back of the body is yang. Your head is yang; your feet are yin. The outside of your arms and legs are yang; the inside is yin. Internally, Qi is yang; blood and body fluids are yin. The five major organs or viscera (liver, heart, spleen, lung, kidney) are yin; their partner organs (gallbladder, small intestine, stomach, large intestine, and bladder), called bowels in TCM, are yang. Because yin and yang have an inseparable relationship, you can see that if there is a problem with one, the other will have one also.

Here's a case study that illustrates this theory very well. One of my patients had had constipation for virtually her entire life. She had tried many natural remedies to help her bowel movements. Her nose was always stuffed up, but she never had a cold. She also complained of skin problems, which she referred to as acne, that appeared during her menstrual cycles. She had changed her diet innumerable times and tried many combinations of natural herbs. Although these attempts helped a bit, she could never entirely get rid of this problem. Immediately, two of her symptoms told me that her lung energy was dysfunctional. Why? Because according to TCM theory, the nose is the "window" or opening of the lung and the skin is the "tissue" of the lung. Both are under this organ's control. These two clues coupled with her constipation and the fact that she couldn't relieve it through diet or herbs, told me that addressing her constipation and the large intestine (the lung's partner organ) was only part of the real problem.

From my classical training and experience, I knew that her lung had to be treated if she really wanted to deal with this problem at its source and cure this condition. I used acupuncture and certain herbs to treat her lung and large intestine at the same time. After four visits, her problem was about 80 percent fixed. I then prescribed several foods such as pears, honey, and almonds that she could eat to help heal her lung completely. Her condition had improved to such an extent that she was now ready to take charge of her own healing and finish the job. Several months later, she called to let me know that her constipation had completely disappeared and her skin had improved dramatically. Interestingly, I see this problem frequently in my practice. Many Western women who have skin problems have no idea that their condition is related to a deeper problem that is a function disorder of the lung and the large intestine. The normal, healthy working relationship of both with each other has been disrupted. I try to educate my patients that if they want beautiful skin, they must be sure that this yin/yang pair works in harmony. Expensive creams and procedures can only address skin problems from the outside. Truly beautiful skin really does come from the inside.

The energies of yin and yang are the basis of the most fundamental method of TCM diagnosis because it sees all disease or imbalances in terms of the Eight Principal Syndromes: yin and yang, interior and exterior, cold and heat, and deficiency and excess. Ideally, yin and yang should always remain in harmony, not, as many people think, in balance. The words balance and harmony are sometimes used interchangeably, but I would like you to understand that in TCM theory, they are quite different. Balance is merely the first step toward harmony. Two things can be balanced; they can have equal weight in a scale and yet still be separate.

Harmony means that they are not just equal, but blended into a seamless whole. This condition of harmony reflects a dynamic state where these energies wax and wane automatically. When one predominates, the other recedes. For instance, when too many days of summer heat build up, nature will cool the earth down with thunder storms. If Indian summer occurs and the weather is too hot, eventually nature will create rainy weather, which will inevitably be followed by cooler days. These same dynamics of yin and yang energies continually occur within your body.

Let's go a little more deeply into this concept. Balance has to do with the relationship between two separate entities: the

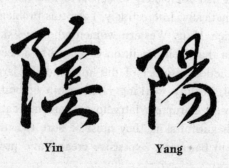

Yin   **Yang**

relationship between you and me, for instance, or the relationship between your heart and your kidney. First, the relationship has to be in balance. Once it's in balance, the next step is to achieve harmony. When two things are in harmony, their energies blend together. Exchanges between things that are in balance have to be "manual," like going to the bank to transfer money from one account to another. When two things are in harmony, there is an ongoing, unconscious dance between them that happens naturally. In other words, you no longer have to go to the bank, or make the transfer in a conscious way. In a healthy system, this "automatic transfer" happens naturally, both within the body itself, and between the body and the outside forces of nature we've already discussed. For example, when nature's energy changes, your internal energy will respond automatically. When the seasons change like summer into fall, your internal energy will readjust itself to match nature's new energy frequency. If you can't make this switch smoothly, then you will catch a cold. That's why so many people get sick when fall arrives. At this time, because fall is related to the lung (whose opening, remember, is the nose), these problems show up specifically as coughs, sneezing, allergies, and loose stool (which relates to the large intestine).

TCM principles teach us that we are not isolated individuals; we are part of the Universe. To get support from the Universe, your body must function at its best: it must be in harmony. Each organ's Qi must be strong, it must function well, and its relationship with all the other organs must be in harmony as well. There are different levels—some high, some low—of balance and harmony. For instance, when you're young and healthy, your body is functioning at a high level of balance and harmony. When you're older, you may not be able to perform the same way you did in your youth, but you can still have a healthy body as long as you maintain balance and harmony.

Let's apply this theory to breast cancer. In TCM, the healthy energy of your body is yang; the unhealthy energy of cancer is yin. If there is enough yang energy, the yin energy of cancer will remain in balance and not affect the body. If the yang energy declines (for whatever reason), then yin energy will begin its rise. Within each person, there is a certain tolerance level or turning point, beyond which yin comes into control. At this moment, when yin becomes stronger than yang, cancer's energy dominates the body. Modern science describes this situation very well in the catastrophe theory. Now, suppose you've gone through chemotherapy and radiation successfully. Your internal energy level will never reach its previous stage because these therapies have damaged it; however, you can bring yin and yang back into harmony within your body, even at this reduced level. And, if you do—through Qigong, foods, meditation and lifestyle changes—according to TCM theory, you can actually prevent a recurrence of cancer. Keeping yin/yang in harmony is the key to a healthy body. TCM believes you always have the power and the potential to be 100 percent the best for your body's system, whatever its limitations.

TCM has an ancient saying: "As long as you know the principle of yin and yang, you can be a good TCM doctor." This sounds simple, doesn't it? Everything is based on yin and yang. This is easy to say, but difficult to understand, and even more difficult to apply as a principle. Many, many classical Chinese medical texts discuss yin and yang theories; yet, you cannot learn this principle from books because they do not say how to use it. You need a guide, someone who has not only knowledge, but also a feeling for the essence of this simple principle. Today, the principle of yin and yang is not really understood very well. Therefore, it is difficult to learn how to practice it. The key to good health is always yin and yang. If you know about this principle, you will have a much deeper understanding of the Five Element Theory, and be able to use its ancient medical knowledge successfully for breast cancer prevention, treatment, and beyond. There is a good example of how one of my patients with breast cancer applied this theory during her radiation treatments in Chapter 13.

THE THEORY OF QI

Qi is vital energy, the animating force of the Universe. It makes up the sun, the moon, the stars, the earth, and all things animate and inanimate. Everything has Qi. There is the universal Qi of the celestial planets, the Qi of seasons, and the earth Qi of time and place. There are two types of human Qi: one you receive or inherit from your parents, the other you build up day by day after birth. Qi is also the means by which all things are connected and can communicate with each other. Although unseen, Qi is every bit as real as other natural phenomena such as wind, gravity, magnetic forces, and the like.

Most of us live our lives without thinking about how information is passed among animate and inanimate systems. Things that may not seem to "talk" with each other, trees, for example, do indeed communicate, and they do it through Qi. People also communicate, not just by talking, but through Qi. For instance, the words "You look great" take on various meanings depending on the Qi, or energy, with which you send them. You may convey enthusiasm, jealousy, or indifference, by the way you use your Qi to send these words. The words are the same; they

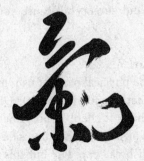

Qi

are merely vehicles that transfer the energy of your meaning. The power of the message lies in your Qi.

Why is Qi Important to Self-Healing and Health?

In ancient times, a good doctor of TCM knew everything about Qi; it was clearly recognized as the essence of TCM. According to the *Nei Jing*, the best doctor knows the "three Qis" of heaven, earth, and humanity. A good TCM doctor also understands that all three are related, that humans are just one part of the overall web of energy that weaves everything in the Universe together.

Within the body, TCM is more concerned with the function of each organ, than with the physical organ itself. As TCM says, "All physical problems emanate from Qi that is out of harmony." For each of your body's organs to function well, their individual Qi must flow freely. Then, for a healthy body, we must go another step: all the organs must work in harmony. TCM uses Qi to describe each organ's function. For example, if you have frequent urination or get up frequently during the night to urinate, it means you have a kidney Qi deficiency. Your kidney does not have enough power to send the right message to your bladder to hold this water until morning. If you have menopausal hot flashes, you also have a kidney Qi deficiency. A chronic back pain can also indicate the same problem. Chemotherapy, radiation, and surgery all cause your body to develop a Qi deficiency.

How Does Qi Work?

When we die, the physical parts of us remain; the only thing that is different is that our life force—our Qi—is gone. Qi gives everything life, without it there is no growth nor change, but this animating force or power is just one side of Qi. Qi is usually translated into English as "energy," but this force is more than energy, it encompasses intelligence and function. Of these forces—power, intelligence, function—the last two are the most important.

Each of your body's organs, for example, has its own Qi, its own function or purpose. Like a television set, your body needs power to operate, it must be plugged into a source of energy. Yet to receive a clear picture—for the body to function well and be healthy—each component has to work well alone. Then it must also work in harmony with all its fellow components. It is important to realize that the malfunction of one single component can affect the operation of the others, as well as the operation of the whole television set.

Your body's organs are like different television channels; each has its own frequency. If the frequency of a channel is wrong—if the organ's function is off in some way—the television can't receive and display a good picture on that channel, no matter how much energy is there. You may be thinking, "but that is only one channel, there are others." Because the function of one organ is related to all the other organs, a problem with one, if left unattended, will ultimately affect the function (the frequency) of the others. There can be plenty of power but none of the channels will be able to receive a clear picture. In a sense, the power of Qi needs the intelligence or function of Qi to give it direction. (This is why, from the TCM standpoint, organ transplants are so difficult to make a success. While the physical organ structure of the donor and recipient may look alike, the Qi of each one and how each functions is very different from body to body.)

TCM is built on this theory of an interconnected whole system linked by Qi with all internal systems (organs) functioning in harmony. TCM understands the nature of things, but only in relation to other things. We could say it is a model of relativity. The description of something is always in relation to something else. This relates to the concept of yin and yang energies outlined above. TCM does not just focus on the mechanics of a thing or problem. For example, in the case of headaches, TCM does not just treat the headache pain (which it considers a symptom), but tries to identify the root cause of the headache.

Seasonal Qi

Most of us live in a world buzzing with physical feedback from noise, smells, sounds, sights, and the like. We run from morning to night at breakneck speed, rarely taking time to see, let alone feel, changes in the weather or the seasons. Yet each season has its own Qi. Nature understands this. For instance, if you plant something out of season, it may grow, but never flower or bear fruit. The plant is responding to the seasonal Qi in which it was planted. Each season's particular Qi allows different things to change. Whether we believe it, or can perceive it, each season's Qi exerts an influence on our bodies and in our lives, as well. Working with the flow of nature can give you added healing support. Often, many people get sick when the seasons change. This is because their bodies' Qi cannot adjust smoothly or match with the Qi of the new season.

TCM has a theoretical framework within which each organ has a seasonal relationship. For example, spring is the season of the liver. It is a time when nature's Qi rises naturally, causing seeds to germinate and plants to grow. In your body, liver energy rises in the spring as well. Each organ is particularly prone to problems during its own season. Spring can bring headaches, especially on top of the head where the liver meridian runs, if liver Qi rises too forcefully. It can also bring on bad moods or mood swings if liver Qi does not flow smoothly. Why? Because your liver is in charge of emotions.

Nature's Qi changes with the seasons. Summer is the season of heat and relates to the heart. Many heart problems have to do with an excess of heat in this organ. Fall energy relates to the lung; its energy can make you vulnerable to coughs and colds. And the season of the kidney is winter, when this organ tends to suffer from problems such as infections and deficient Qi. Weak kidney Qi is one reason why you may feel especially tired and low during the winter. To follow nature's law during seasonal changes, you should nurture or support your yang energy during the spring and summer. For example, at this time, you can eat shrimp to increase yang energy. During the fall and winter, you should support your yin energy. For instance, TCM has certain kinds of herbs that are good to take at this time of year.

Organ Qi

Because TCM sees the human body as a microcosm of the Universe, if each season has its own Qi, then so does each organ. This special Qi helps each organ to function properly; it carries the special messages and information that causes the organ to perform its natural job. Without its Qi or animating force, the organ is dead. For example, the Qi of the liver naturally rises and spreads out freely. As we've seen, this quality helps the liver perform one of its main functions—ensuring the smooth flow of both Qi and blood throughout the body.

In your body, the organs communicate with each other via Qi and the meridians. For instance, if your liver is not well or out of balance, it will tell its "sister" organ, the gallbladder, which will then tell the stomach, and so on. Internally, you are a very busy switchboard abuzz with constant messages about the state of your health! If an organ's Qi is excessive or deficient, an organ function disorder will result; however, these disorders will be different. For instance, if a person has a stomach and spleen Qi deficiency, you will see pale lips and a fat tongue with a white coating. This will usually be accompanied by cold hands and feet. This person often has diarrhea and a poor digestive system. If a woman, she may have vaginal discharge, a lengthy period, and may bruise easily. She may also have cellulite.

If a woman's stomach has an excess of Qi—either caused by itself or the liver—you might see that the tongue has a yellow, greasy coating. She may have bad breath and stomach distention and experience constipation. Sometimes the nose becomes very red. Or, she might have tempromandibular joint (TMJ) and bleeding gums. Many times, my women patients are surprised at the root cause of their stomach problems. Usually, they tell me "No one's ever told me this. I just had a battery of tests and my reports show that everything is okay." I explain to them that being angry and under a lot of stress causes a liver function disorder. In this case, the flow of their liver Qi has been disrupted. It has become stuck in the stomach, the organ it controls. Then the liver generates excessive heat. When this happens, these women experience stomach pain, distention, acid indigestion, etc. They tell me that they've tried everything to treat their stomach. I tell them that the real problem lies in their liver function and that unless this is treated, their stomach problems cannot heal.

Qi and Blood: Intertwined Rivers of Life

In TCM theory, blood is the "mother" of Qi; it carries Qi and also provides nutrients for its movement. Qi is the "commander" of the blood. This means that Qi is the force that both makes blood flow throughout the body and guides it to the places it needs to be. Blood and Qi affect one another and are inseparable. We can use the principle of yin and yang to describe these two vital elements. Blood is yin; Qi is yang. Without the yin energy of the physical blood, the formless Qi has no place to reside. On the other hand, without the yang energy of Qi, blood has no life force. While one cannot survive without the other, they also have control over one another. Within this relationship, blood and Qi have the dynamic ability to transfer various properties back and forth.

If your Qi is deficient, you will also have deficient blood

and vice versa. For instance, spotting between menstrual cycles, if there is no tumor or internal bleeding, is seen by TCM as a serious sign that your Qi is deficient. In this case, because Qi is deficient, it cannot do its job of making sure blood flows normally. If blood is deficient, the body's internal environment will not be balanced nor well-nourished. After childbirth, for example, women sometimes experience a low-grade fever. From the TCM point of view, this is caused by blood deficiency, not an infection. TCM would counteract this condition by increasing a woman's Qi or increasing her blood through special herbs and foods. For this condition, ginseng is one of the best herbs to reduce fever and increase Qi. TCM would not prescribe antibiotics, because it does not believe the source is an infection. Deficient blood can also play a part in other problems, such as various other menstrual disorders, heart palpitations, and insomnia, to name a few.

Problems stemming from deficient Qi can cause a lot of physical discomfort and distress. Because these are energy problems, when they occur, they are usually beyond scientific measurement. Yet, you may feel uncomfortable all the time, suffering from symptoms such as headaches, bad moods, poor digestion, and insomnia. Frequently, Western medical tests cannot find anything wrong. Certain problems may appear, or worsen, at specific times of day. This has to do with the daily cycle of Qi among the twelve organs. Each organ has a two-hour period when its energy is at its most responsive to internal and external factors. For the lung, for instance, this time is from 3:00 A.M. to 5:00 A.M. If you find yourself waking up between these hours, perhaps with a cough, it could be a sign that your lung Qi is weak or deficient. This is an energy problem— again beyond scientific measurement. A good TCM practitioner can immediately recognize the condition as an energy-based one and begin the proper treatments to help you heal it. (See the

Self-Healing Checklist for Sleep Habits in Chapter 15 for a list of hours when each organ's Qi is on duty.)

The condition of deficiency can be debilitating. You can have a deficiency of overall Qi or you can have a deficiency of a specific organ's Qi. In either case, it means that the thing in question has insufficient power to do its proper job. Deficient Qi, especially of the kidney, is a very serious matter. Of the two main types of Qi—the one we're born with (stored in the kidney), and the one we build up after birth—most of us unwittingly drain our irreplaceable kidney energy far too much. We keep drawing on our energy "savings account" that is stored in the kidney. Instead, we should be drawing on our energy "checking account," which is accumulated through the stomach.

As your kidney energy account gets low, problems begin to show up in other areas, starting in your weakest organ. When Qi is deficient, the entire body stops functioning properly. If this happens, you may experience a number of uncomfortable symptoms, yet your medical and scientific tests might still be normal. At this time, you should become alert to the fact that your organs are sending you an "SOS"; they are basically saying, "Help! We're not playing in harmony any more. We're falling out of balance!" This is the time to take preventive actions to safeguard your precious energy system; this is not a time to ignore the internal messages your body is sending. Often, women with deficient Qi are told that there is no physical basis for their complaints and discomfort. TCM sees things very differently.

Here's an interesting example of how one organ's Qi deficiency can spread to another organ and cause the same problem. Several years ago in the middle of winter, a woman in her late thirties came to me with a cough that had persisted for more than three or four months. She had tried a number of different doctors, many cough medicines, and several antibiotics. She was becoming desperate in her effort to get rid of this constant cough. Most debilitating was the fact that the cough kept her up almost every night. Nothing could completely relieve her cough. At the same time, she also complained of urinary frequency, lower back pain, and weakness in her knee joints.

TCM has a unique way of evaluating a cough, which it considers among the most serious of conditions and among the hardest to treat. Its medical theory states that each organ can cause a cough; a cough doesn't only come from the lung. My challenge was to discover as quickly as possible which organ was causing this woman to cough. I combined a pulse diagnosis with her specific complaints, as well as an understanding that winter is the season ruled by the kidney, and confirmed that the root cause of her cough was definitely a kidney Qi deficiency. In the Five Element Theory (which we'll discuss in deeper detail shortly), the kidney is considered the child of the lung; conversely, the lung is the mother of the kidney. When the child experiences a Qi deficiency, it will draw Qi from its mother and cause the mother organ to develop its own Qi deficiency. This is typical of a classical Five Element case called "The Child Steals Energy from The Mother." My patient's Western treatments targeted her lung problem; they didn't address the actual source of her problem. I prepared a special formula that helped my patient increase her kidney Qi and relieve her lung cough. This treatment addressed both the urgent symptom and the root cause simultaneously. After one week, her cough improved by about 80 percent and she was able to sleep through the night. This helped her healing ability to recharge itself. After the second week, her cough stopped completely.

THE FIVE ELEMENT THEORY

The Five Element Theory, like yin and yang, appears deceptively simple; however, it reflects the entire Universal law in one complete, comprehensive system of related categories of

CLASSIFICATION OF THINGS ACCORDING TO THE THEORY OF THE FIVE ELEMENTS

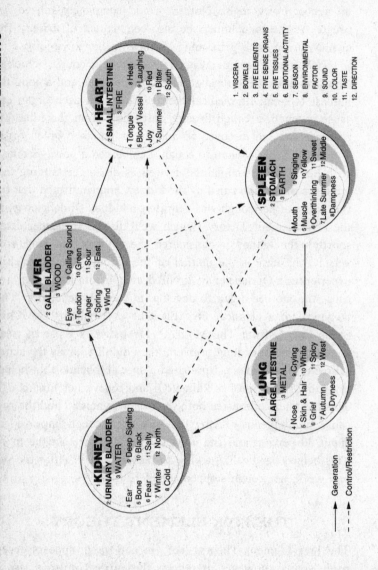

1. VISCERA
2. BOWELS
3. FIVE ELEMENTS
4. FIVE SENSE ORGANS
5. FIVE TISSUES
6. EMOTIONAL ACTIVITY
7. SEASON
8. ENVIRONMENTAL FACTOR
9. SOUND
10. COLOR
11. TASTE
12. DIRECTION

1 HEART
2 SMALL INTESTINE
3 FIRE
4 Tongue 8 Heat
5 Blood Vessel 9 Laughing
6 Joy 10 Red
7 Summer 11 Bitter
12 South

1 SPLEEN
2 STOMACH
3 EARTH
4 Mouth 9 Singing
5 Muscle 10 Yellow
6 Overthinking 11 Sweet
7 Late Summer 12 Middle
8 Dampness

1 LIVER
2 GALL BLADDER
3 WOOD
4 Eye 9 Calling Sound
5 Tendon 10 Green
6 Anger 11 Sour
7 Spring 12 East
8 Wind

1 LUNG
2 LARGE INTESTINE
3 METAL
4 Nose 9 Crying
5 Skin & Hair 10 White
6 Grief 11 Spicy
7 Autumn 12 West
8 Dryness

1 KIDNEY
2 URINARY BLADDER
3 WATER
4 Ear 9 Deep Sighing
5 Bone 10 Black
6 Fear 11 Salty
7 Winter 12 North
8 Cold

→ Generation
--→ Control/Restriction

things. The ancients of Chinese medicine understood that all things were subject to the natural law. Today in Western society, we have forgotten this simple truth. Man is, indeed part of nature. He is not separate or apart from it. Nor can man control nature. Many of the problems we see now, not only in health-care, but in the environment, are related to our thinking about our role in nature. Besides understanding that everything is connected, TCM also learned how to apply this principle of connect-edness thousands of years ago.

Each element of this comprehensive theory—wood, fire, earth, metal, and water—is at the center of a web of relationships that link categories of other things. These are not man-made categories, but reflections of nature's laws. These relationships extend throughout the natural world. Each element, for example, corresponds with a season, a climate, a stage of growth and development, a color, an organ, a tissue, and an emotion, among other things. I urge you to study the Five Element Theory chart on page 84. According to TCM, all aspects of the human body and mind are also related by their nature to one of the five elements. This includes not only the principal organs—liver, heart, spleen, lung, and kidney—but every other part of the body, including emotions, and the five aspects of the soul.

Although described in many medical textbooks, most Westerners are not aware that the Five Element Theory goes deep into Chinese culture where it forms the foundation of disciplines like Feng Shui, the I Ching, and the martial arts. This powerful theory, unfortunately, is gradually fading out of practice because many practitioners would prefer to rely on science instead of its seemingly simple wisdom. The essence of the Five Element Theory has all but been lost. Part of the reason is that the ancient people who discovered this theory had a very different connection with nature than we do today. They were able to tune in to things on a deep energetic level that is almost impossible to do in our overstimulated world. They also understood that nothing in the Universe lives a separate life. The Five Element Theory encompasses the two dynamic relationships of generation and control that connect the five major organ systems. Generation means that one organ is the mother of another organ. Control means that one organ acts as a feedback system for its organ partner and keeps it functioning smoothly, neither excessively nor deficiently, neither too strongly nor too weakly.

GENERATION: MOTHER AND CHILD RELATIONSHIPS

ORGAN	Liver ⇨	Heart ⇨	Spleen ⇨	Lung ⇨	Kidney ⇨
GENERATION	Mother	Mother	Mother	Mother	Mother

The Five Elements themselves are also not inert substances. They are fundamental energies in nature, and they are always in motion. Each element generates, or gives birth to, another. These element pairs are known as mother and child. Each element also restrains or controls another. The right amount of control keeps all the elements in proper proportion. This kind of interaction enables all the elements—all the organs—to work in one harmonious system. If their relationships are good, you are healthy; if any of the relationships become unbalanced, you will suffer from health problems. This is the way the body really works.

Let's see how this Five Element Theory applies to a real life problem. Take your digestive system, for example. To have good digestion, your liver must exert the right amount of control over your stomach. Too much or too little control both create a problem. Experiencing too much anger, or anger over a long period, will impair your liver's proper function (as we have said a number of times, the emotion of anger is related to the liver; excess anger throws this organ out of balance) and cause your liver Qi to overcontrol your stomach's function. Their relationship will then be disrupted. You may suffer from constant abdominal distention or indigestion; you may burp a lot and have a sour taste in your mouth (sour being the taste associated with the liver).

We've seen what happens when the liver overcontrols the stomach and spleen. Now, look what happens when the liver is deficient or too weak to exert the proper amount of control over the stomach. You might experience poor digestion; you might have loose stools, your stomach might become distended after you eat, and if you eat too much cold food or dairy products, you might feel stomach pain. Or, you might start gaining weight. These problems may also interrupt normal sleep habits. What appear to be stomach problems, in reality, originate in your liver.

One of my patients complained to me that every day, at a specific time, she would get a stomach pain and then get diarrhea, after which she would feel better. I felt very bad for her because this problem had gone on for more than five years. She had been to most of the important medical centers at universities throughout the East. After many, many scientific tests, not one doctor could identify her problem, much less offer her relief. Some suggested her problems were mental in origin. From her pulse diagnosis and the description of the time frame of her problem, I knew it was related to a Qi imbalance. I was able to tell her that her liver and stomach relationship had become disrupted and that her liver was overcontrolling her stomach. Because she was suffering from a function problem and not a physical one, her medical tests were unable to identify or recognize what was wrong. To fix this kind of problem, it is essential to fix the liver. So, I developed a special combination formula of herbs to help the liver and stomach relationship rebalance itself. After drinking this herbal combination for one week, her longtime problem completely disappeared and did not return.

Here's another example of the Five Element Theory at work. Your kidney and its healthy functioning is of the utmost importance. It is crucial to understand its role as the source of support for all your organs. A strong kidney supports its "child," the liver. Strong kidney function is essential also to restrain the "fire" of the heart. Sometimes the influence of the kidney is hidden behind the relationship between other organs. For example, the fire of the heart—excess heat in this organ—must control the lung, which corresponds to metal. If the heart has too much fire, the lung will also overheat, causing problems with its corresponding tissue, the skin. But let's track down the true source of this excess heat. Where is it really coming from? The heart may have too much fire because the kidney is not strong enough to restrain it. So the dry, itchy skin that nothing seems to relieve may actually have its root cause in deficient or weak kidney Qi.

Over time, if you hold too much anger in your body and have more stress (the late-twentieth century disease!) in your life than you individually can deal with, Qi, your life force, will become stuck somewhere in your body and eventually create heat. This is true of any excessive emotion. Anything that doesn't flow, that remains stuck or stagnates, generates heat much like a compost heap. Different emotions affect different organs. We now have seen how anger and stress, as well as frustration and depression, affect liver function.

To understand why this information is so critical to helping heal breast cancer or prevent it or a recurrence, remember we said that the liver is the most important organ for women's health. Now, add to this fact that the left side of your body is controlled by your liver. Add to this information another key fact: the liver's meridian runs up to just below the breast area. According to TCM, stagnating Qi in your liver meridian, or unbalanced liver function, can lead to breast cancer. When applied to health problems, the Five Element Theory is indeed complex, yet it provides the knowledgeable TCM practitioner with a unique framework within which diagnoses can go deeply into the problem. Treatments can do more than cover up symptoms. This fundamental theory allows TCM to view the body from the holistic viewpoint; its sophisticated feedback system demonstrates how unbalanced elements can upset the delicate workings of the whole organism.

The twelve meridians control human life, yet they are also the place where disease can live. If disease starts in the meridians, the physician can use the meridians to treat the root cause of the disease.

Therefore, the good physician must start by learning the basic theories of meridians. The advanced physician ends by delving into the endless complexity of meridians. The mediocre physician regards the meridians as simplistic. The best physician regards the meridians as the most complicated system of the human body.

NEI JING (475-221 B.C.)

THE THEORY OF MERIDIANS: UNDERSTANDING THE BODY'S AMAZING ENERGY NETWORK

Your body has twelve major meridians or energy pathways. Each one is related to a specific organ. The earliest records describing these pathways date from between 722 B.C. and 221 B.C. TCM believes that the meridians (sometimes called "channels") form an energy network that covers the entire body. They link with each other and connect all structures and all parts of the body—skin, tendons, bone, internal organs, cells, atoms—as well as connect the interior with exterior and the upper body with the lower body. This interlinked, animating network through which Qi flows freely allows the body to function as an organic whole.

You can think of the meridian network as a collection of highways, roads, and streets that links major cities. The highways (meridians) and the cities (organs) make up an entire energy map (your body). It is over this collection of roadways that energy (Qi) runs. For a better understanding, let's take this analogy further. If a city's internal streets are blocked with traffic, eventually this situation will cause a problem with the highways leading into this city. If the traffic condition worsens, even the cities linked by the major highways will experience a problem. Or, suppose two cities are fine and traffic is flowing smoothly within their areas. If there is an accident and traffic builds up on one of the roads linking the cities, eventually one or both of these cities will find themselves affected by traffic congestion. This is a way to understand how blockages in your meridians can cause problems with your organs.

Meridians form a powerful information system within which each organ also operates its own data system. Your body is constantly communicating with itself. In addition to sending Qi, meridians also transmit actual information to and among your organs. The various body parts communicate with each other faster than the speed of light, sending an incredible array of signals—signals to make certain chemicals, signals to turn up your thermostat, signals that your body is ready to release water, and much more—traveling over this network every second of your life. Meridians are also sensitive to time. They reflect and respond to the changing energy of the seasons and time of day. When your meridian system functions well, your body is healthy and maintains that dynamic condition of internal harmony we talked about in the section above on yin and yang energies.

Meridians form the passageways through which Qi travels

throughout your body. The ancient medical text, *Nei Jing,* states: "The function of the channel (meridian) is to transport the Qi and blood and circulate yin and yang to nourish the body." Because meridians respond to and carry stimulation as well as transmit information, they have the ability to bring healing energy to various parts of your body, affecting physiological and other changes as Qi circulates. It is this function that makes acupuncture and acupressure work; the flow of Qi in the meridians can be enhanced or modified either with needles or with the pressure of the finger or the hands.

The understanding of these energy pathways and the organs they link provides TCM with a framework for pinpointing the root cause of health problems, as well as the diagnoses to heal them. Meridians work by regulating the energy functions of your body. They help coordinate your organs' work and keep your body balanced. If a dysfunction occurs, acupuncture or other therapy can be used to further stimulate the relevant meridian(s) to bring an affected organ back into balance. If Qi stagnates for too long in any meridian, the Qi can become blocked up and eventually turn into matter—conditions for a physical mass can then occur. Also, if a meridian suffers from a dysfunction, it becomes susceptible to outside disease factors that can eventually make their way into your internal organs along the route of the affected meridian. TCM theory states that as long as Qi flows freely through the meridians, the body can avoid disease. Practicing the *Wu Ming* Meridian Therapy movements in this book can help you keep your Qi moving smoothly through the meridians running through your breast area.

CRITICAL MERIDIANS RELATING TO BREAST CANCER

Six bilateral meridians run through the breast area: stomach, liver, kidney, lung, pericardium, and spleen. Qi, or vital energy, can stagnate in any of them. More than 50 percent of breast cancers are diagnosed in the area of the breast where your stomach meridians run. The other areas of the breast where cancer develops relate to your kidney and liver meridians. Twelve percent of breast cancers appear in the areas where each of these meridians run. Other organs account for the rest of breast cancer diagnoses. Your breast can have a problem with one or more of these meridians—either singly or in combination. Simple multiplication then tells us that there are 720 different types of Qi stagnation conditions that can create breast problems ($6 \times 5 \times 4 \times 3 \times 2 \times 1 = 720$).

Meridian theory is complex. Let's look at where these critical energy pathways run in your breast area. This will help you comprehend how complicated problems are that develop in the breast area and how vital it is to keep Qi flowing freely in these six critical meridians. This will also help you understand the root cause of breast cancer and how to address it. Let's take a look at each meridian and its location. These bilateral meridians follow the paths described here. They also have other deep internal branches that connect them with their respective organs as well as other organs, the sense organs, and various structures of the body. Meridians form an amazing energy network that reaches into every part of the body.

BREAKING CANCER'S ENERGY PATTERN

According to TCM meridian theory, if the stomach meridian's Qi stagnates in the breast area, then your breast cancer will show up in the outer, upper quadrant or on the center line that runs through the breast. If your kidney meridian's Qi stagnates in your breast area, then your cancer will appear in the inside upper quadrant. If your liver meridian's Qi stagnates in the breast area, then your cancer will develop in the outer, lower quadrant. Eighty-five percent of breast cancers occur in these three areas. Keeping your Qi running smoothly in these three major meridians can dramatically increase your chances of controlling the development of breast cancer, or its recurrence. Keeping your Qi running smoothly in these three critical meridians can also help keep your Inborn Qi, which resides in the kidney, strong and your whole body functioning in harmony. When this happens, you can help yourself avoid cancer's energy pattern—even with a genetic or inherited predisposition for this disease.

To follow are descriptions of the path that these six meridians take on the left side of body:

The Stomach Meridian

This meridian begins internally at the side of your nose and emerges in its first acupoint under the eyes. It runs down to your chin then separates into two branches: one follows the jaw line and rises to the forehead near the hairline; the other descends along the side of your neck and then runs down through the center of your breast area in line with the nipples. It then jogs inward and drops straight down to the lower stomach. The meridian then runs down the outside of your thigh and lower leg. When it reaches the middle of the ankle it runs on top of the foot to end at the outside tip of the second toe.

The Liver Meridian

This meridian starts at the base of the nail inside the big toe. It rises along the bones of the big toe, on top of the foot to a point just above the inside anklebone. It then runs up the middle of the inside portion of your lower leg and all the way up the inner thigh to the vagina area. The liver meridian makes a circle around the vaginal area. It then runs up the side of the abdomen to the free end of the eleventh rib and ends at the point between the sixth and seventh rib bones just under your breast.

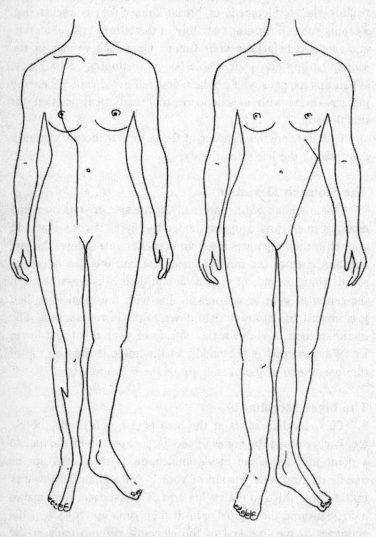

Stomach Meridian   **Liver Meridian**

For women, the liver meridian also has one extra branch that runs inside the body and stops at the nipple. Classical TCM theory states that the left side of the body is controlled by the liver; the right is controlled by the lung. A woman's breast area in general is controlled by the stomach meridian and the nipple itself is controlled by the liver meridian. It's apparent then that both meridians need to function smoothly to avoid Qi stagnation or worse.

The Kidney Meridian

This meridian starts at the underside of your little toe. It runs crosswise to the center of the sole of the foot, then up across the instep to the area around the inside anklebone. From there it rises behind your liver meridian along the inside back of your leg, then up the back of your inner thigh. From there it moves internally through the vertebral column and eventually reemerges just above the pubic bone. It travels up the abdomen just off the centerline of the body. As the kidney meridian approaches the breast area, it jogs outward slightly (further away from the body's centerline), runs up through the breast and ends just below the collarbone.

The Lung Meridian

This meridian starts on the lateral portion of your chest (near the shoulder) in the space between the first and second ribs. It then travels down the inside of the arm (in line with the thumb), passes through the wrist, and ends at the outside corner of your thumbnail (on the radial side).

The Pericardium

This meridian begins in the breast area just to the outside of the nipple (in the fourth intercostal space). It moves up and out through the shoulder and down the middle of the inside of the arm (traveling between the lung and the heart meridians).

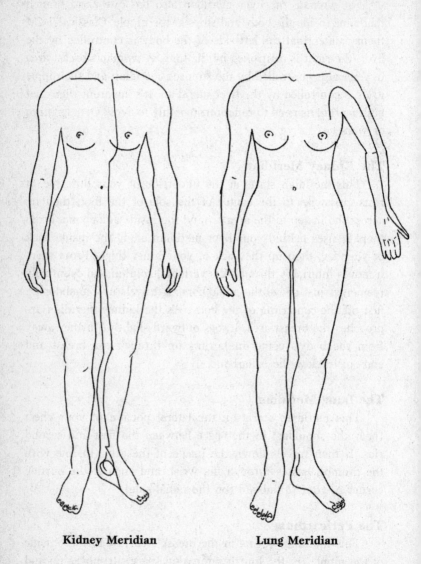

Kidney Meridian   **Lung Meridian**

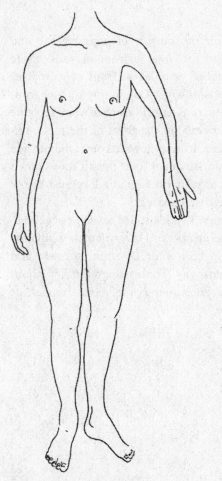

Pericardium Meridian

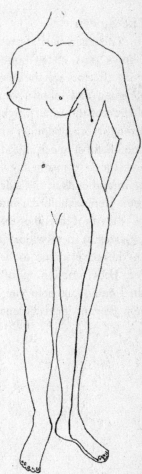

Spleen Meridian

Moving through the wrist it travels through the center of the palm and ends at the tip of your middle finger.

The Spleen

This meridian starts on the outside of your big toe and follows your instep bone to the area in front of your inside ankle. It runs up the inside of your leg in front of your liver meridian and follows your shinbone. Continuing up the front portion of the inner thigh, it runs up the front of your hipbone through your abdomen and rises up the front of the torso outside of the stomach meridian. It then flows through the outside breast area to just below your shoulder joint then it drops down again and ends at the side of your rib cage at a level just below your nipple (the sixth intercostal space).

Based on meridian theory, I've identified seven special healing gates in these major meridians. You can stimulate acupoints on these meridians to help keep your Qi running freely and your body functioning in harmony. These energy gates, if stimulated daily, can help you reduce your risk of breast cancer, or help prevent its recurrence.

CHAPTER 7

How Your Body's Five Major Organ Systems Function Individually and as a Whole System; What Happens When Relationships and Communication are Disrupted in Breast Cancer

WHEN TCM talks about an organ, its definition is broader than that of Western medicine. In TCM, the term "organ" refers not only to a physical structure, but also to a holistic complex of functions both physiological and psychological. In addition to its function in the various systems of the body, each organ also governs a body tissue and a sense organ (the organ's "opening"), is related to a particular emotion, and houses one of the five aspects of the soul. These functions are all closely interrelated and can have a strong effect on one another. TCM views each organ in this fuller context. Throughout this book, I have used the classical reference, which is singular for both kidney and lung.

Each organ is especially susceptible to its ruling emotion. As mentioned earlier, chronic anger (as well as frustration, depression, and of course, stress) can actually affect the way your liver functions. Conversely, a liver problem or disease can, in turn, cause anger, or frustration, or depression, and stress. While your organs have a physical connection with each other, equally important, TCM understands that they also have an energetic or Qi connection. This energy relationship can be direct or indirect. Organs that have no physical connection with each other, for instance your lung and large intestine, share a very important Qi connection through the relationship of their meridians. Your lung also has an important Qi connection with its "child," the kidney, and with the liver, the organ that it controls. Western medicine tends to see only the physical, scientific relationships among your body's organs. TCM has an ancient medical framework within which your body's inherent Qi-based connections fit.

The good news is that both medical systems are moving toward each other in interesting ways. Western medicine, for example, is proving scientifically that your stomach is related to your brain, and can have a powerful effect on what goes on there. Recent research has uncovered the way epithelial cells in the stomach's lining communicate with the brain—a scientific window on "gut feelings." TCM has understood this Qi connection for thousands of years. The stomach is considered the "child" of the heart, and the heart is the organ that controls all mental activities. TCM treats all mental problems by treating the stomach—healing the "child" through its "mother." Although they've arrived at the same understanding, TCM uses Qi to understand the human body; Western medicine works within the physical paradigm.

THE LIVER AND ENERGY FLOW

In the Five Element Theory, the liver's partner organ is the gallbladder. Its element is wood. The opening gate to the outside of the body is the eye. The tissue it controls is the tendon. The emotion that can affect the liver is anger. The seasonal energy and time that matches the liver is spring. Its environmental factor is wind. The color related to liver Qi is green. The taste

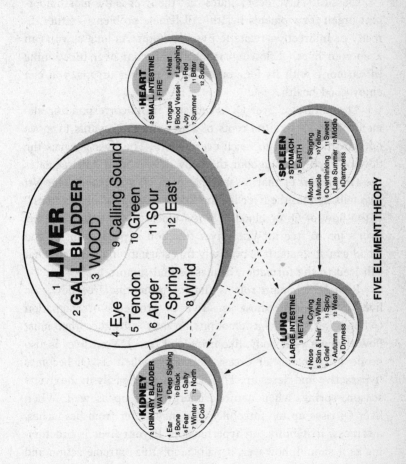

FIVE ELEMENT THEORY

1 HEART
2 SMALL INTESTINE
3 FIRE
4 Tongue
5 Blood Vessel
6 Joy
7 Summer
8 Heat
9 Laughing
10 Red
11 Bitter
12 South

1 SPLEEN
2 STOMACH
3 EARTH
4 Mouth
5 Muscle
6 Overthinking
7 Late Summer
8 Dampness
9 Singing
10 Yellow
11 Sweet
12 Middle

1 LIVER
2 GALL BLADDER
3 WOOD
4 Eye
5 Tendon
6 Anger
7 Spring
8 Wind
9 Calling Sound
10 Green
11 Sour
12 East

1 LUNG
2 LARGE INTESTINE
3 METAL
4 Nose
5 Skin & Hair
6 Grief
7 Autumn
8 Dryness
9 Crying
10 White
11 Spicy
12 West

1 KIDNEY
2 URINARY BLADDER
3 WATER
4 Ear
5 Bone
6 Fear
7 Winter
8 Cold
9 Deep Sighing
10 Black
11 Salty
12 North

that goes directly to the liver is sour. The direction or location is East.

Classical TCM theory states that the liver is the most important organ for women's health. All female problems—either directly or indirectly—relate to liver function. As long as you can keep your liver Qi flowing smoothly and your liver functioning in harmony with its four other major partner organs, you can enjoy good health.

The nature of liver Qi is reflected in its corresponding element of wood: like the roots of a tree, liver Qi wants to move outward freely and to reach everywhere. The liver governs the flow of energy throughout the body. It smoothes and regulates the circulation of that inseparable pair: Qi and blood. The *Nei Jing* tells us that the liver is "the Root of stopping all extremes." If the flow of Qi or blood becomes blocked or stuck, it is your liver's job to free it. When liver function is poor, your Qi and blood can stagnate. It is precisely this stagnation, over time, that can lead to the formation of masses and tumors.

Because its main role is that of promoting free flow, the liver is the organ most sensitive to problems of stagnation (whether of Qi, blood, emotions, or any substance that must flow through your body, like urine and feces). Your liver is also prone to problems of excess, especially when its Qi becomes hyperactive and flares up. This happens most easily in the liver's season, spring, when nature's energy rises up as well. When liver Qi rises up too forcefully, you may suffer from headaches, dizziness, irritability, or hypertension. If your liver is functioning as it should, however, it will "stop" this extreme action and relax the excessive flow of Qi that is moving too strongly.

In the TCM paradigm, any problem that occurs on the left side of your body is related to a liver dysfunction. If you always get a headache on your left side, or your left nostril is always stuffed up, or your left shoulder has a pain, or you notice a weakness in your left ankle, or you always fall on your left side or bump into something on your left side, then you should recognize that your liver is not working properly. Even if all your scientific tests are normal, you definitely need to work at healing your liver. A well-trained TCM doctor would recognize this problem immediately.

Once I had a patient who had suffered from migraine headaches for a great many years. She had been to both Western and Eastern doctors. No one could help her relieve her terrible pain. Every month before her period, she would get a headache that would start on the left side of her head. Before it came, she would see an explosion of light on the left side. After I did a pulse diagnosis, we sat down to talk. I told her that her three symptoms—headache before her period, headaches starting on the left side, and the light on her left side before her headache— gave me very strong clues. I told her these were significant signs pointing to a serious liver function disorder. Because she had had this problem for so long, I advised her that she needed the kind of herbs that needed to be cooked, she needed acupuncture, and she needed to change her lifestyle. It turned out she was a teacher and experienced a great deal of constant stress. Her treatment time was longer than most patients. Finally, I was able to help her totally relieve her migraine headaches and PMS. Later, she called me to let me know not only was she well again, but she had just had a beautiful baby!

LIVER AND SPLEEN: A SERIOUS PARTNERSHIP

Your liver has an important relationship with your spleen, particularly because they share responsibility for maintaining good digestion. If your spleen does not get the proper support from your liver, it will not be able to transform food into the life-sustaining elements of Qi and blood. Your liver, which stores your blood, depends, in turn, on your spleen to provide an adequate supply of nutrition. Deficient liver blood shows up especially in those areas of the body that correspond with the liver's element of wood: your nails, eyes, ligaments, and tendons. Dry, cracked, brittle nails are one sign of deficient liver blood, so are dry or burning eyes. Vision also relates to the liver; problems with liver Qi can cause vision to blur or deteriorate. Because your eyes are the "opening" of the liver, the reverse is also true: too much "looking" hurts the liver. Overuse of the eyes—for instance, long hours in front of your computer—can actually drain liver Qi.

One day, an attractive business woman in her mid-thirties, in pretty good health, came to my office complaining that her left eye had been burning and had hurt for about six months. She had tried a number of over-the-counter remedies and had seen several ophthalmologists, but her problem persisted. Her pulse diagnosis told me that her condition was being caused by liver Qi stagnation. In the "asking" part of my examination, I asked her whether she had anything sad or distressing happen to her six months ago. She told me that just about that time, she had had a very difficult divorce that produced tremendous anger and resentment in her. She felt, however, that she had dealt with it and had put her emotions to rest. She acknowledged that it was then that her problem had started. Once we identified that the source of her eye problem was coming from an excess of liver heat, we were able to develop a plan that included acupuncture and herbs. We also talked about the fact that the root cause was her excess and unrelieved anger. To fix her problem, we then discussed a number of ways that would help her let this anger go. Within three weekly visits, her pain virtually disappeared. Although her symptoms were alleviated, I told her that she could only heal completely if she worked at rebalancing her liver's energy with certain foods and lifestyle changes. Above all, she had to find a way to let her negative emotions go. This woman really wanted to get completely better, so she made a number of lifestyle and emotional changes that over time healed her problem.

People experience anger when someone has done something negative to them directly, or they interpret a given set of circumstances as being directed at them, whether this is true or not. Sometimes anger or resentment is deep-seated and difficult to let go of. You can help yourself, by training yourself to take a step back and look at a situation from a different angle. You might find surprising things happen. For example, suppose you love your boyfriend and do everything to help him through law school. Now, he has graduated with your help and he has become very successful. He finds a new girlfriend and leaves you. This is definitely a cause for anger. Your emotion is appropriate, but you can't let it destroy your life and your health. If you can take a step back, you can see that if he stayed with you, he might also have broken your heart by cheating. You may have spent more years with him than you cared to. This way you should consider yourself lucky so that you are now free to find someone who will truly love you. I really want everyone who reads this book to understand that anger and stress can directly affect your liver function. When your liver function becomes unbalanced, you can get sick. TCM understands that long-term anger and resentment can cause serious health problems. Don't let other people and outside situations make you sick. The following tips can help reduce anger precisely because they cause something to break that, in turn, helps relieve a Qi blockage.

TCM Tips for Relieving Anger

Here are three, time-tested ways to release anger.

- Find a safe place and break several glass bottles.

- Buy a dozen (or more!) eggs and smash them.

🐌 Scream as loud as you can (your shower or your car are good places to do this!).

Some menopausal women suffer from joint pain, and this, too, relates to the liver, which governs tendons and ligaments. Proper joint function depends on sufficient blood from your liver to nourish tendons and ligaments. Interestingly, many people, especially women, do not realize that overexercising can harm their liver and tendons. Excessive aerobics and excessive jogging, for example, are both very bad for your tendons. These problems can be prevented by using moderation. Women who overexercise or run too much, are unwittingly depleting their liver Qi. Often, they find that their periods stop. In extreme cases, excess exercise can cause chronic fatigue syndrome. To conserve Qi for healing, I recommend that my patients who have undergone chemotherapy or radiation avoid strenuous exercise. I give the same advice to my many menopausal patients.

LIVER AND BLOOD: ONE OF THE MOST IMPORTANT PARTNERSHIPS FOR WOMEN'S HEALTH

The liver's role in regard to blood is especially important for women. A properly functioning menstrual cycle depends on the liver to regulate the flow of blood (as well as store it). If your liver Qi becomes unbalanced—either too much or too little—symptoms like PMS, irregular periods, headaches, cramps, and distending pain in the breasts will occur on a regular basis.

In the West, most of us would not think to connect these symptoms with the liver. Yet, such problems are the norm for many women who suffer through difficult menstrual cycles year after year. They don't realize that these debilitating conditions are symptomatic of a deeper internal imbalance that their own bodies can resolve, if given the proper support. Ignoring these internal warning signs can put a woman at risk for breast cancer.

If you are menopausal or postmenopausal, a smoothly functioning liver is essential to good health. Even after your period stops, the proper circulation of Qi and blood is just as vital to good health. Because the liver's function is sensitive to so many energy changes (such as seasons, emotions, weather, and the like) and is related to so many organs, managing emotions to keep liver Qi flowing smoothly is crucial for women of all ages in the prevention of breast masses and cancer.

Uterine cancer also relates to your liver. Although the liver meridians do not pass through the uterus itself, everything having to do with this organ depends on the healthy function of the liver and proper flow of its Qi. Stagnant Qi and blood due to poor liver function can cause the formation of hard lumps, masses, and tumors, such as uterine fibroids and ovarian cysts. If prolonged and severe enough, Qi stagnation or the blockage of Qi can lead to cancer.

LIVER, UNBALANCED EMOTIONS, AND STRESS: ROOT CAUSES OF BREAST CANCER

TCM views the high incidence of breast cancer in Western society as liver Qi stagnation caused by prolonged stress and emotional excess—especially anger and overthinking. Just as your liver's job is to keep the flow of Qi and blood running smoothly, it also must keep your emotions flowing evenly as well. Poor liver function can show up in its corresponding emotions of anger, depression, and stress, or in a more general feeling of uneven moods, like frustration, irritability, or nervous tension.

If you suffer from a liver function imbalance, you will become frustrated easily and your emotions may tend to get blocked and stuck. You might have trouble unwinding from the day's tensions. You may also have difficulty, like the patient I just described, in letting things go. You may use your energy and emotions to dwell on the same issues or problems over and over. Some of the things you think about may have occurred long ago, but you still let them use up your precious vital energy in the present. And while poor organ function can cause emotional problems, the reverse is more often the case. TCM believes your emotions are very powerful energies that affect the way your organs function. A poorly functioning liver can have a profound effect on your whole body, especially in relationship to the organs with which it has important partnerships. The liver and stomach pair is one good example; the relationship between your liver and your heart is another. It is impossible to overstate the importance of reducing stress in your life. Stress goes right to your liver where it can either cause or aggravate many problems: from migraine headaches to high blood pressure, to insomnia, to menstrual and digestive problems. Stress is more than a daily annoyance. According to TCM, it can be the root cause of life-threatening conditions. We've seen how TCM theory states that the left side of the body is controlled by the liver, and we have seen that the area of the nipple also falls under the liver's control. Its meridians run through the breast. Given the fact that the left breast is more vulnerable to breast cancer than the right, you can see why it is crucial that the liver's function remains healthy. Managing your emotions and making a concerted effort to lower your stress level is essential to the prevention of breast cancer or its recurrence.

TCM'S Top Ten Problems That Reveal How Well Your Liver is Functioning

- ❦ Brittle fingernails

- ❦ No half moons on nails

- Eye irritation

- Tendon problems

- Migraine headaches, especially on the left side

- Anger or unstable emotions

- Stress

- Indigestion and bloating

- Menstrual problems/PMS

- Yeast infections

THE HEART AS KING

In the Five Element Theory, the heart's partner organ is the small intestine. Its element is fire. The opening gate to the outside of the body is the tongue. The tissue it controls is the blood vessel. The emotion that can affect the heart is joy. The seasonal energy and time that matches the heart is summer. Its environmental factor is heat. The color related to heart energy is red. The taste that goes directly to the heart is bitter. The direction or location is South.

TCM considers the heart the king of all the organs. "If the king is happy, there is peace and harmony in the kingdom." While your kidney provides the power for your whole organ system, your heart's job is to provide the soul. Every organ needs Qi to function; it also needs the right message or organizing soul force. These messages come from your heart. Your heart animates all the organs, maintains their proper function, and enables them to come together and act in concert—like one grand symphony of exquisite harmonics. Your heart, as well as your liver, also performs an aspect of controlling the circulation

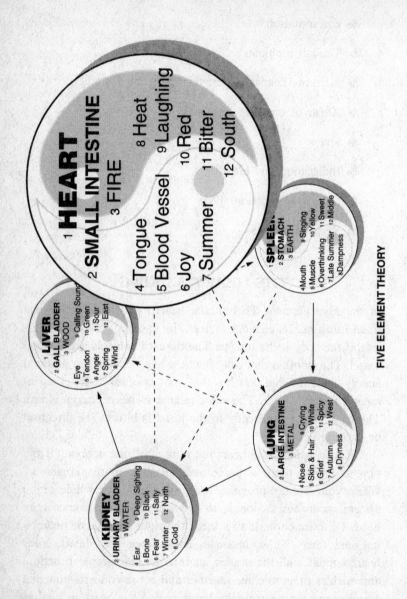

FIVE ELEMENT THEORY

1 HEART
2 SMALL INTESTINE
3 FIRE
4 Tongue
5 Blood Vessel
6 Joy
7 Summer
8 Heat
9 Laughing
10 Red
11 Bitter
12 South

1 SPLEEN
2 STOMACH
3 EARTH
4 Mouth
5 Muscle
6 Overthinking
7 Late Summer
8 Dampness
9 Singing
10 Yellow
11 Sweet
12 Middle

1 LIVER
2 GALL BLADDER
3 WOOD
4 Eye
5 Tendon
6 Anger
7 Spring
8 Wind
9 Calling Sound
10 Green
11 Sour
12 East

1 LUNG
2 LARGE INTESTINE
3 METAL
4 Nose
5 Skin & Hair
6 Grief
7 Autumn
8 Dryness
9 Crying
10 White
11 Spicy
12 West

1 KIDNEY
2 URINARY BLADDER
3 WATER
4 Ear
5 Bone
6 Fear
7 Winter
8 Cold
9 Deep Sighing
10 Black
11 Salty
12 North

of blood. The heart has another assignment; it controls different aspects of your mind and emotions than that of the liver.

More than any other organ, your heart must have strong kidney support. Palpitations, for example, are a signal that your heart lacks the support of sufficient blood or Qi. If you experience palpitations, your heart is not getting enough blood. And there isn't enough Qi or energy to help keep blood flowing smoothly. Consequently, your heart must pump more forcefully to keep blood moving. Strong Qi is essential to good circulation. As we know in the West, heart disease surpasses breast cancer when it comes to killing women. Why does heart disease affect so many postmenopausal women? The reason, from the TCM standpoint, is that menopausal women who develop heart disease already have a kidney Qi deficiency. To effectively treat this problem, TCM believes it is essential to increase kidney Qi, which in turn, will reestablish the delicate relationship between these organs. (The heart's natural element of "fire" must remain in harmony with the kidney's natural element of "water.") For thousands of years, TCM has understood that the key to longevity lies in keeping the marriage of this special pair a harmonious and happy one.

Unless there are physical defects in the heart or arteries, heart problems often have their root cause in weak kidney function. We've mentioned women who reach menopause. Older people, too, are more susceptible to heart problems because kidney Qi declines naturally with age. During our later years, the kidney has less Qi to do its proper job of cooling the heart or controlling its fire. Very simply, your heart will overheat if your kidney is too weak to cool it down. Your heart also controls body fluids. TCM says "perspiration is the liquid of the heart." If you perspire too much and too often, your heart may have a Qi deficiency problem, or conversely, this excessive loss of fluid can cause a Qi or energy deficiency of the heart. You may want to rethink your exercise routine, especially if it makes you perspire too much. By trying to improve your cardiovascular health, you may actually be impairing it. According to TCM, sweating too much is definitely not a good thing; neither is excessive exercising. Once in a while, we are shocked by the death of a younger athlete who succumbs to a sudden heart attack. If exercise is supposed to help protect the heart, then why do these seemingly healthy people die?

Because excessive internal and external heat can give your heart problems, it has a special guardian in the form of the pericardium. The pericardium defends your heart and also helps to keep it from overheating. Different kinds of Qi or energy stagnation can cause the heart to overheat. Some signs of an overheated heart are a dry mouth, thirst (especially at night), cold sores, and yellow urine. Also, your skin may break out; you may even suffer from nightmares. In extreme cases, an overheated heart can result in mental illness. Heart fire can also affect your digestion. The heart and small intestine share a close energy connection. An overheated heart can pass its fiery Qi through the meridians to your small intestine, which plays an essential role in absorbing nutrition from food. Too much heat in your small intestine can interfere with this ability to extract nutrition. The result is poor digestion. This can make your body feel uncomfortably full, or produce that infamous symptom—heartburn!

The heart also shares another close energy relationship with the liver, its "mother." When your liver is overstressed, its Qi is drawn elsewhere and cannot support your heart's work. Your liver not only supplies your heart with blood, it plays an important role in circulation, ensuring that the flow of your blood is smooth and steady. In TCM theory, the three major organs having to do with blood are the heart, liver, and spleen: the heart controls blood circulation, the liver stores blood and regulates its flow, and the spleen creates both Qi and blood from the essence of food. The spleen also helps the liver by keeping blood flowing within the vessels. This intricate web of connections keeps your whole body functioning smoothly.

The cause of some heart problems can be difficult to pinpoint. According to TCM, high blood pressure can, for example, be related to the heart, the kidney, or the stomach. As always, this ancient medical system is not so much interested in the symptoms, but wants to identify which of these organs is the source of the problem. With high blood pressure, the root cause, generally speaking, lies with a combination of organs. High blood pressure is not a simple problem because it comes from the functional disorder of multiple organs. When you suffer from this condition your entire body is out of balance—the whole building needs work! This type of imbalance brings us back to the key principle of yin and yang. The flow of each of these energies should follow its natural direction: yang Qi naturally rises; yin Qi naturally descends. This does not happen with high blood pressure. Too much Qi goes up, where it gets stuck in the head. To treat high blood pressure, TCM treats the overall imbalance in the body's energy system and works to get the whole body back in harmony.

High cholesterol and clogged arteries are other examples of function problems whose origin can reside in several organs. Most often, their root cause is in your liver. When any or all of the organs function poorly, your body gradually loses its self-regulating capabilities and falls out of balance. (When your body is well, it manages cholesterol levels very nicely and keeps your arteries open.) This is true even if the organs themselves are fine physically. The body becomes inefficient and sluggish. Substances such as fat, water, and toxins tend to accumulate. It is vital, at this point, to identify why your body is falling out of harmony. In other words, TCM will still search for the root cause, rather than just treat the symptom.

Complex problems such as high blood pressure or high cholesterol do not receive disease-specific treatment from TCM. In fact, TCM does not even categorize these problems in Western medical terms. A good TCM doctor will analyze a patient's individual symptoms; diagnosis and treatment will focus on the organs determined to be the root cause. In contrast, Western medicine might approach this condition by trying to suppress or control its symptoms with medication. It will tend to isolate or divide the problem into parts and treat the parts. For instance, the side effects from taking high blood pressure medication may be offset with additional drugs. These drugs, in turn, can cause their own side effects, and so on. TCM does not separate a patient from his or her symptoms, it views the person as an integrated whole. It always looks at the larger picture of the body's energy system, as well as its relationship with the Universe. Its goal is to get your whole system back into balance. Over millennia, TCM has developed a vast body of experience and knowledge that has led to a singular understanding that a body in balance has the ability to heal itself.

As king of all organs, the heart houses the *Shen* or spirit. It also houses the control center for the other four aspects of the

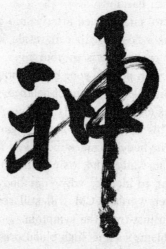

Spirit

soul, which reside in the lung, spleen, liver, and kidney, according to traditional Chinese understanding. TCM considers your heart to be the ruler of all mental activities. When TCM speaks of the mind, it has a broader meaning than that in the West. It includes aspects of consciousness in the concept of "mental activities": intelligence and thinking; memory and sleep; emotions; as well as the various aspects of the soul. In TCM's view, most mental and sleep problems can be traced straight to the source—unbalanced heart Qi. Because the heart relates specifically to intelligence, TCM recognizes that meditation can be applied to help relieve emotional distress.

TCM also has a different view of the function of blood: it not only nourishes and moistens your body, it is the material basis for all mental activity. Normal mental activity depends on good blood circulation and sufficient blood supply. Your heart itself relies on strong Qi and adequate blood to house your spirit. If your heart is weak or overheated as described earlier, or if it is not supplied with enough blood, your spirit cannot rest peacefully there. Often, with this problem, your whole body may feel uneasy and restless, thinking may be cloudy, and memory poor. Insomnia and nightmares may occur. Have you ever had a night when your mind seems to float? You feel you are asleep, yet you're aware of being awake at the same time? TCM views this as an indication that your heart is unable to "house" your *Shen* or spirit. If you want to feel calm, think clearly, and sleep soundly, you must take care of your heart. Above all, if you can keep your heart in a joyful, peaceful state, you can also help reduce the effect of stress on the all-important liver. Consequently, you can also help heal breast cancer and protect yourself against it or a recurrence. What can you do to take care of your heart? Work at keeping all your organs functioning in harmony. Try not to overuse your mental faculties. Try to maintain a positive, happy outlook at all times. Many patients find this hard to believe, but the most powerful exercise I can recommend is the following: face the mirror and smile at yourself . . . really smile at yourself, from your heart. This is very difficult for most people to do, but if you can smile from your heart, not just a fake smile, you will help make the blood and Qi flow throughout your whole body. Then try smiling at others from the heart. Smiling from your heart can make a big change in your physical health. This is one kind of special Qi-gong exercise.

THE SPLEEN AND THE STOMACH: YOUR ENERGY CHECKING ACCOUNT

THE SPLEEN: YOUR ENERGY GENERATOR

Dr. Li (1180 to 1251 B.C.) is considered the first physician in Chinese history to develop the theory of the prominence of the stomach. He is acknowledged to be the most famous specialist on the functioning of this organ. His wisdom puts it this way: "All human health problems are initially caused by a spleen/ stomach dysfunction."

In the Five Element Theory, the spleen's partner organ is the stomach. Its element is earth. The opening gate to the outside of the body is the mouth. The tissue it controls is the muscle. The emotions that can affect the spleen are overthinking and anxiety. The seasonal energy and time that matches the stomach is late summer. Its environmental factor is dampness. The color related to spleen energy is yellow. The taste that goes directly to the spleen is sweet. The direction or location is Middle.

Proper functioning of the digestive system depends on the spleen, which, with its partner, the stomach, is the body's main source of energy after birth. You can think of them as being linked into one "checking account." It is from this account that

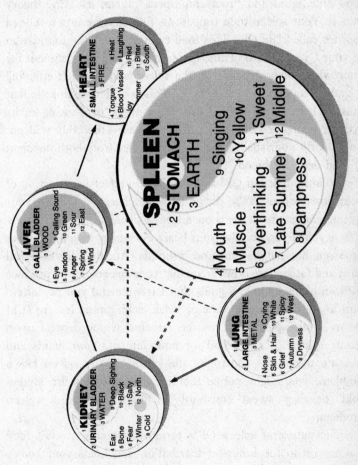

FIVE ELEMENT THEORY

1 HEART
2 SMALL INTESTINE
3 FIRE
4 Tongue
5 Blood Vessel
Joy
8 Heat
9 Laughing
10 Red
11 Bitter
12 South

1 SPLEEN
2 STOMACH
3 EARTH
4 Mouth
5 Muscle
6 Overthinking
7 Late Summer
8 Dampness
9 Singing
10 Yellow
11 Sweet
12 Middle

1 LIVER
2 GALL BLADDER
3 WOOD
4 Eye
5 Tendon
6 Anger
7 Spring
8 Wind
9 Calling Sound
10 Green
11 Sour
12 East

1 LUNG
2 LARGE INTESTINE
3 METAL
4 Nose
5 Skin & Hair
6 Grief
7 Autumn
8 Dryness
9 Crying
10 White
11 Spicy
12 West

1 KIDNEY
2 URINARY BLADDER
3 WATER
4 Ear
5 Bone
6 Fear
7 Winter
8 Cold
9 Deep Sighing
10 Black
11 Salty
12 North

the body's daily energy expenditures should be drawn. It is where the body gets the Qi to create food and liquid. TCM refers to this energy as "Acquired Qi." Your stomach receives food and liquid and "rots and ripens" them, as TCM theory puts it. Your spleen then transforms this mixture into a refined essence called "*gu* Qi." This food essence forms the foundation of your Qi and blood. Thus, the daily fuel and nourishment for your whole body depends on the spleen and stomach enjoying a healthy cooperative partnership. This is a lifetime linkage that must be kept strong. If their function is weak, or if eating habits become poor—or both, as is often the case—the body will not be properly nourished. Then you can suffer from both deficient Qi and deficient blood.

Because deficient Qi has the ability to affect the function of your other organs, TCM puts a lot of emphasis on keeping your spleen and stomach in good shape. Deficient blood not only affects your liver, but also your heart. As we have seen, it causes problems like palpitations and insomnia. Anemia, dry skin and hair, and fatigue are other signs that your spleen cannot produce sufficient blood. Other signals that I recommend you pay attention to are poor muscle tone or weak, aching muscles. In TCM theory, your spleen governs the muscles, which depend upon strong spleen Qi and blood for nourishment. Your hands and feet are under the control of the spleen. If the spleen has a problem, you might notice that these extremities are always cold, or they sweat constantly. Cellulite is also a spleen problem.

The nature of spleen Qi is to move upward: it sends food essence up to the lung for distribution and holds your body's organs and tissues in place. A weak spleen cannot perform these functions. Spleen problems tend to be ones of deficiency—the spleen seldom suffers from problems of excess. When your spleen Qi is so weak that it sinks instead of rises, prolapse of your organs can occur, especially of the stomach, intestines, uterus, and rectum. Other symptoms of weak, sinking Qi are diarrhea, fatigue, and blurred vision. Your spleen plays an important part in the transportation not only of food essence, but also of fluids throughout the body. A weak spleen does not have the power to properly regulate all the fluids in your body, which can lead to excessive dampness. Your spleen definitely does not like dampness because it interferes with its function of transforming and transporting your nutritive essence. Poor spleen function can cause a range of digestive problems: lack of appetite, poor digestion, loose stool or diarrhea, and abdominal distention. It can also cause you to retain water and gain weight.

Weight is a very big issue in the West. If you have trouble losing weight, the problem may be your spleen. Look at your tongue: if it is fat, with a thick white coating, it is a signal that your body is unable to rid itself of excess water. I tell my patients to be careful about trying to lose weight. Dieting can make the problem of ridding your body of excess water worse because it can weaken your spleen Qi further. Even if you lose weight, you're apt not only to gain it back, but also to have even more trouble losing it again. Overeating is not the cause of this extra weight; it is a function disorder. In the Dragon's Way, my Center's self-healing weight loss program, I concentrate on improving the functions of the spleen and stomach and helping this all-important partnership come back into harmony. When this happens, the body loses weight naturally. You cannot lose this weight by dieting, because you must increase the body's Qi, not decrease it, which is why so many diet programs fail. You also have to learn how to eat for healing—to avoid cold foods such as salads and raw vegetables, for example. (See the Self-Healing Checklist on Eating Habits in Chapter 15 for more information relating to the care of the spleen and stomach.)

The spleen controls the flow of blood, how it flows, where it flows and how much blood should flow into a given body structure. Remember that the liver also relates to blood circulation, its interest is in storing blood and making sure it flows freely. It has no interest in controlling where the blood flows. It just keeps the blood moving. If the spleen has a problem, there will usually be conditions of internal bleeding. A woman with poor spleen function may experience an abnormally long menstrual cycle or spotting between periods. The tone and elasticity of blood vessel walls is also the spleen's job. If it is too weak to perform this function, your blood vessel walls may become fragile and even collapse. This can cause bruising, varicosis (a varicose condition of the veins), and chronic bleeding.

A lot of menopausal women suffer from frequent spotting and excessive bleeding. In the West, hysterectomy is one of the biggest solutions to this problem. It is, however, something I recommend avoiding, if possible. Removing the uterus takes away an extra organ, or engine, that provides the body with a special source of Qi. According to TCM, excessive bleeding does not originate in the uterus or ovaries, but in deficient spleen Qi. This organ is too weak to control the blood and its flow through the blood vessels. Fixing this problem means going to the source and fixing the spleen. Surgery will not do this; it can, in fact, make matters worse by damaging important meridians and weakening the body's overall Qi.

My Western patients are very surprised when I discuss the root cause of excessive bleeding and I tell them TCM has thousands of years experience treating this condition successfully. Often, only a few treatments produce excellent results. In my practice, I use special herbal formulas adapted specifically for my Western patients and acupuncture to help women stop this kind of bleeding and save their uterus in the process. Naturally, this is very important to my patients in their child-bearing years. It also helps them avoid future problems when they enter menopause.

While your heart houses the *Shen*, your spleen offers a home to the *Yi*—the aspect of the soul that provides the capacity for applied thinking, concentration, and some functions of memory, particularly long-term. Too much thinking or worry (the spleen's corresponding emotion) can deplete your spleen's Qi. They can also lead to depression, one of the major twentieth century problems. Depression is frequently treated with drugs like the popular Prozac and many others. Often these antidepressants can cause side effects that affect the stomach. A lot of my women patients ask me if TCM has a way to help alleviate depression because they want to discontinue these drugs. My response is that they must fix the underlying spleen condition first. I advise them to consult their doctors before stopping any medication. Then, together we work out a plan to treat the spleen by changing the patient's diet; identifying negative lifestyle habits that can be improved; and using acupuncture to help the liver function more smoothly. There is also one classical Chinese formula in use for centuries that I have adapted for my Western patients. This combination of treatments has proven highly effective in the treatment of depression.

In many women, excessive thinking and worry are also coupled with poor eating habits, thus delivering a double blow to a smoothly operating spleen/stomach partnership. Long before a woman reaches menopause, her spleen may have been weakened substantially, resulting in many of the symptoms outlined above. TCM does everything possible to save the spleen if it has a problem. It believes that this organ plays an essential role in an individual's overall well-being. You will see when we discuss the stomach below how this information relates to breast cancer and its prevention.

Ancient TCM Tip For Self-Healing

Spices prescribed to help relieve cold and damp energy in the spleen and stomach:

- Cinnamon

- Ginger

- Fennel seeds

- Garlic

- Black and white pepper

- Chinese barley (from a Chinese food store)

THE STOMACH

TCM considers your stomach a bowel; that is, it fills up with food and water, digests and transforms these materials, then empties itself. TCM places tremendous importance on stomach Qi. It is sufficient stomach Qi that helps all five major organs to operate in a healthy manner; a deficiency can lead to weakness in all of these organs. As we've seen, a properly functioning stomach working in cooperation with your spleen supports the daily activities of your body. According to TCM theory, whether or not your body can recover from illness or disease depends on a strong stomach/spleen partnership. This has vital importance to those with breast cancer or undergoing cancer treatment.

From my experience, stomach problems, either of deficiency or excess, are always connected to liver function problems. These two organs share a control relationship and the liver will strive to keep this relationship in balance. If the stomach suffers from a Qi deficiency, then naturally, digestive problems will follow. Here are a few signs that will help you identify a Qi deficiency. You often feel a dull pain in your stomach; if you are hungry or fatigued, your pain increases. Eating warm foods, taking a rest, massaging your stomach when fatigued relieves your pain. You experience stomach bloating and loose stool; you have a fat tongue with a white coating and your hands and feet feel cold. If you experience pain and you rest, the problem goes away. If massaging your stomach or eating something warm helps relieve the pain, then generally speaking, your condition is one of deficiency. In the case of a Qi deficiency, make sure you avoid cold food and cold fluids, as much as possible. Stomach Qi deficiency can also cause hypoglycemia and migraine headaches. In this case, the migraine headache will usually occur across the front of the forehead, which is where the stomach meridian runs.

If, on the other hand, your stomach suffers from a condition of excess heat, then you will experience a different set of problems. Liver energy will stagnate in the stomach causing burping, rib and stomach distention, and stomach pain. Often there will be a sour taste (associated with the liver), or persistent bad breath. The tongue shows a yellow or even a red coating. You may even be continually constipated. If these conditions occur, it is important to treat the liver as well as the stomach, otherwise the root cause of the problem remains. Often this excess heat comes from emotional problems such as anger and stress. It can also be caused by fried foods, spicy foods, and excess alcohol. This condition too can cause a migraine headache, in the front of your forehead. TMJ and gums that bleed or swell are related to excess stomach heat. The reason is that the stomach meridians run through these areas and are connected to these structures.

The nature of your stomach is warmth-loving. What does this mean? It means that the ancient doctors were able to tell that the natural law, as it applies to the stomach, indicates that this organ "dislikes" cold energy and cold essence. Just as plants have a natural environment within which they grow and thrive, so do our organs. We can't take indoor plants and grow them outside in climates that are too harsh. Nor can we force hardy outdoor plants to grow for us inside our heated homes. These organisms act according to an innate natural law that is appropriate for them.

Let's go back to the stomach and its natural law of loving warmth. Continually fed a diet of cold food, uncooked food (like raw vegetables or salads), or cold fluids (like ice water and soda), your stomach's function can become unbalanced or suffer from the Qi deficiency symptoms described above. This might cause stomach distention, stomach pain, an overweight condition, loose stool, and even migraine headaches. If your stomach's dysfunction produces constant symptoms like these, this is an indication that your stomach meridians are also encountering problems. This can be quite serious. If Qi stagnation of the stomach meridians occurs in the breast area, there is a risk that eventually breast masses and even breast cancer can occur. Studies have shown that 50 percent of breast cancers develop in the breast area where the stomach meridians run. I cannot stress strongly enough how vital it is to keep Qi flowing smoothly through this meridian. As we've said, according to TCM, chemotherapy and radiation can seriously unbalance the stomach's proper functioning. This is why so many patients experience nausea, loose stool, lack of appetite, and other symptoms during these types of treatments. I usually prescribe a combination of TCM herbs and special herbal teas to help relieve the side effects of breast cancer treatment. Information on TCM herbal combinations and teas for breast cancer can be obtained from our Traditional Chinese Medicine Foundation, whose address is in the back of this book.) For those who want to prevent breast cancer or its recurrence, paying attention to keeping this all-important pair well is vital. Women undergoing breast cancer treatments will find that these treatments are particularly destructive of stomach/spleen Qi. I urge you to work with the checklist of eating habits in Chapter 15, as well as the healing foods listed in Chapter 17.

BREAST CANCER, BREASTFEEDING, AND THE STOMACH MERIDIAN

The La Leche League of Schaumburg, Illinois, has a Center for breast feeding information. In their *Facts about Breastfeeding 1997*, they cite a number of studies that relate to breastfeeding and human milk providing protection against a variety of cancers. One discusses the slight reduction in the risk of lymphomas observed among children breastfed as infants versus those who were not. Another study shows data about the cancer-preventive effect of breastfeeding to the offspring when their mothers consume soy foods. There is also indication that this might protect the individual throughout life. Women who have ever breastfed had a reduction in breast cancer risk. Postmenopausal women also showed a significant decrease in breast cancer risk with duration of breastfeeding with their second live birth.

This correlates with the TCM point of view. Breastfeeding can make a major contribution to good health and breast cancer prevention because TCM believes that in order to produce enough milk, your stomach must function well. Breastfeeding also gives the entire breast area an energy and physical tuneup because of the stimulation involved. If you can't produce milk, there are a few easy things you can do to help yourself.

Here is one ancient formula for help producing breast milk. Take 3 ounces of peanuts, 3 ounces of soy beans, and 2 pieces of pork feet. You can add a few pieces of orange peel and 2 tablespoons of wine (any kind). Bring all ingredients to a boil, then simmer for one hour. It will become almost like a soup. Eat the peanuts and soybeans, and drink the soup. This ancient recipe can produce results quite rapidly.

THE LUNG:
BREATHING THE BREATH OF LIFE

In the Five Element Theory, the lung's partner organ is the large intestine. Its element is metal. The opening gate to the outside of the body is the nose. The tissues that it controls are the skin and body hair. The emotion that can affect the lung is grief or sadness. The seasonal energy and time that matches the lung is autumn. Its environmental factor is dryness. The color related to lung energy is white. The taste that goes directly to the lung is pungent or spicy. The direction or location is West.

One of your lung's primary functions is the control of your whole body's Qi. From its high position in the chest, your lung governs both the formation of Qi, which occurs within the lung, as well as the distribution of Qi throughout the body. Inhaled air combines with food essence sent to your lung from the spleen, its "mother," or energy-generating organ. The resulting *zong* Qi, which is kind of a master Qi, then becomes the basis for other types of Qi, which are sent like messengers traveling throughout your body to nourish, moisten, warm, and protect it. All of this happens, of course, in less than the blink of an eye during the "automatic transfer" process of the healthy body we discussed in the theory of yin and yang energy in the previous chapter.

Wei Qi (or defensive Qi as it is known), for instance, is dispersed by the lung to the area between the muscles and skin to warm and guard the body's surface. TCM believes that external pathogens such as wind, cold, and heat invade the body through the skin. Your skin is your first line of defense and it is your lung's job to keep this protective mechanism working well. Weak lung Qi impairs this protective function and leaves your body vulnerable to a variety of problems, including increased susceptibility to colds and flu. This may be particularly apparent to you if you always get sick in the fall, the season that the lung rules.

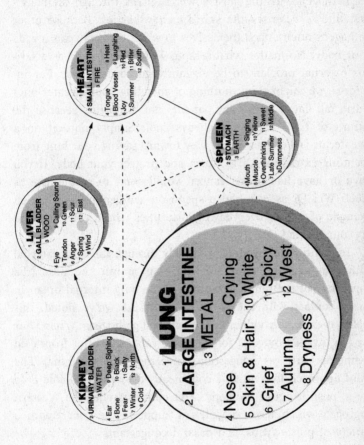

FIVE ELEMENT THEORY

HEART
2 SMALL INTESTINE
3 FIRE
4 Tongue
5 Blood Vessel
6 Joy
7 Summer
8 Heat
9 Laughing
10 Red
11 Bitter
12 South

SPLEEN
2 STOMACH
3 EARTH
4 Mouth
5 Muscle
6 Overthinking
7 Late Summer
8 Dampness
9 Singing
10 Yellow
11 Sweet
12 Middle

LIVER
2 GALL BLADDER
3 WOOD
4 Eye
5 Tendon
6 Anger
7 Spring
8 Wind
9 Calling Sound
10 Green
11 Sour
12 East

KIDNEY
2 URINARY BLADDER
3 WATER
4 Ear
5 Bone
6 Fear
7 Winter
8 Cold
9 Deep Sighing
10 Black
11 Salty
12 North

LUNG
2 LARGE INTESTINE
3 METAL
4 Nose
5 Skin & Hair
6 Grief
7 Autumn
8 Dryness
9 Crying
10 White
11 Spicy
12 West

One way to conserve lung Qi is to dress warmly as the weather becomes cooler in the autumn. Windy days should be regarded as an enemy of good health because wind is the external pathogen with the most power to break through the body's first line of defense—the skin's energy barrier. Because other pathogens often attach themselves to wind, they too, can invade your body. No matter what season, TCM views wind as a serious external problem to be vigilantly guarded against. For instance, you might think nothing of shedding your sweater on a warm fall day. I advise my patients not to do this because the nature of fall's energy is always cool. Simply putting on a sweater or jacket goes a long way toward saving your lung from spending extra *Wei* Qi to warm and protect your body. If you have or have had breast cancer, you'll want to accumulate as much Wei Qi as possible to spend on self-healing. This is an example of finding everyday opportunities where you can build up your healing Qi.

In addition to invading your body through the skin, external pathogens can also enter through your mouth and nose (the "opening" of the lung). Your lung is the only internal organ in direct contact with the exterior world. As we've noted, this makes it extremely vulnerable to external pathogens. When your lung is invaded by cold, for instance, you may suffer from cold symptoms such as congestion, sneezing, and coughing. The TCM approach to treating a cough caused by external cold is to try to push it out of the body. This contrasts with the Western approach which tries to "kill" or suppress the cough with a variety of pills, syrups, and nasal decongestants.

Here's an interesting example of what can actually happen when a cough gets suppressed. I had one patient who is a graphic designer in his late thirties. He came to me to try and cure a terrible skin problem on his hands and arms. The condition, which looked very bad, made everyone afraid to shake hands with him. If he handed over money, people were reluctant to take it. The fluid released by scratching his hands would often cause his girlfriend to have an allergic reaction. By the time I saw him, he had had this condition for more than ten years. He had been to many dermatologists and taken many internal and external remedies; nothing helped.

At first, I used certain TCM treatments to treat it as a usual skin condition. Although this helped somewhat, his skin condition continued to come and go. Then, I asked him if he could recall what happened in his life before the skin condition appeared. He related that he remembered having a severe cough for a few months for which antibiotics were prescribed. When his cough stopped, his hand started to develop a kind of eczema. He could actually remember the first site of this skin problem, which I recognized immediately as an area on the lung meridian. Using my TCM background, I diagnosed that the cough's energy was trying to break out of the body through its skin. I told him that we were going to change his herbal formula and that he might experience a cough. I told him not to worry about this cough because we would be allowing this old problem a way out of his body. As I knew he would, he began to experience the cough we talked about. In just a few weeks, however, his long-time skin problem began to show remarkable improvement. We continued this treatment for a few months. His hands and arms healed completely. This was about five years ago and the problem never returned. This case is a perfect example of how TCM theory can pinpoint the root cause of a difficult health problem. Without a deeper understanding of this ancient medicine, however, I must admit the treatment might seem a little strange.

THE LUNG AS MANAGER OF QI AND NUTRITION

TCM sees the lung as the "manager" of Qi and nutrition. We've seen how your spleen performs its job of sending the essence or Qi of food upward to the lung. We've also described above how the lung, in turn, parcels this Qi out to the other organs. Good digestion is vital to this process, as is eating good quality food. Your lung also plays a part in promoting the circulation of blood. While your heart controls your blood vessels, your lung helps create the energy to push blood through them. If your lung is weak, circulation will be poor, and your body will not be properly warmed and nourished. Symptoms of insufficient lung Qi include cough and shortness of breath, cold limbs and hands, sweating, and fatigue. Your lung is also a key player when it comes to your body's metabolism of water. It directs your body's water downward to the kidney and urinary bladder for elimination. A weakened lung can cause urinary problems or water retention (if you tend to be overweight, it may be a lung problem). And because your lung has a close energy relationship with the large intestine, constipation and diarrhea can also have their origins in poor lung function.

THE LUNG AND YOUR LUMINOUS SKIN

Part of your lung's job as the manager of nutrition is to send fluids to your skin to nourish and moisten it. According to the Five Element Theory, your skin is the body tissue governed by your lung; the condition of the skin mirrors the strength and quality of this organ's Qi. Deficient lung Qi can manifest itself in dry, rough, itchy skin.

What about wrinkles and other signs of aging that show up in the skin, especially in the face? One of the purported benefits of taking estrogen is that it reduces signs of aging, especially wrinkles and crow's feet. TCM, however, has its own understanding of the aging process. TCM relates skin condition not just to your age, but to the quality of lung energy and the level of the body's overall Qi.

All yang meridians (large intestine, triple warmer, small in-

testine, bladder, gallbladder, stomach) converge in the head.
They either begin or end in the face. A Qi or energy problem
in any one of these energy channels—or a combination of
them—can show up in your face. According to TCM, wherever
there are wrinkles, there is an insufficient amount of nourishment and Qi to support muscle and skin health. Having a facelift
cuts through vital meridians and may damage them beyond re-
pair. It's like cutting off the roots of a tree. You may look better
initially, but it's almost inevitable that some unwanted problems
will develop later.

TCM views the face, especially the eyes, as the mirror of
the heart. Remember your heart is home to the *Shen* or spirit;
your face mirrors this aspect of your soul. TCM believes that if
your soul changes, your face will too. This is why TCM's holistic approach concentrates primarily on reducing the signs of
aging from the inside out. External treatment may offer some
benefit, but there is nothing as powerful (or as attractive!) as
letting good health shine from within. The lung is also home to
the *Po,* the physical aspect of the soul. TCM believes this soul
stays in the earth after death. The *Po* controls all your physical
and mental activities. This includes all senses, such as smelling
and hearing, and all movement, whether of your limbs or your
thoughts. Your lung is like the assistant who carries out the
orders of the chief executive; anything that requires movement
depends upon your lung Qi functioning smoothly. Your lung is
also the first organ to die. Because the lung is in control of all
of the Qi that you have built up after birth, when this critical
organ expires, so do you.

Remember that we said that each of the twelve meridians
is "on duty" for two hours at a time in the body. The lung is
the first organ "in charge." Its hours are from three to five
o'clock in the morning. If you continually wake up during this
time period, especially with a cough, you most likely have deficient lung Qi. In other words, when it comes time for your

body's energy to switch from one "commander" to another, you cannot make this transition smoothly because the organ on duty, in this case the lung, is too weak to take over the job. It is not surprising then that most hospital deaths are recorded during three to five o'clock in the morning. Individuals who are critically ill simply do not have enough lung Qi to go on. If they can weather this crucial time period, however, it means that their body has enough Qi or energy to fight another day to try and heal itself.

If you want to prevent breast cancer, you should take good care of your lung. You can see that a function disorder of this organ can disturb the liver, the organ it controls, and the kidney, the organ that is its child. A function disorder can disrupt the delivery of nutrition throughout the body and disturb the healthy functioning of the skin. If you do not have breast cancer and you still smoke, you are definitely disrupting healthy lung function. You may be lucky and remain at this stage for a while. Your physical organ may show no problems in scientific tests, but the way it's handling its job may eventually break down.

Another important influence on your lung is the emotion of sadness. If you find yourself in a chronic state of sadness, please be careful. This is the key emotion with the power to cause a lung function disorder. For those women fighting breast cancer, chemotherapy and radiation will burn up a lot of your body's fluids and will cause a buildup of excess heat. These treatments can also cause a lung Qi deficiency that will manifest itself as fatigue, dry skin, skin breakouts, constipation, or even a cough. I have developed a list that includes a number of foods and herbal recipes in Chapter 17 that you can add to your diet during breast cancer treatment that can help strengthen your lung function.

Ancient TCM Tip For Self-Healing
Six foods you can add to your diet to increase lung Qi:

- Almonds

- Pears

- Persimmons

- Honey

- Lily bulb (from a Chinese food store)

- White mushrooms (not the American kind, but from a Chinese food store)

THE KIDNEY: YOUR ENERGY FOUNDATION

In the Five Element Theory, the kidney's partner organ is the bladder. Its element is water. The opening gate to the outside of the body is the ear. The tissue it controls is the bone. The emotion that can affect the kidney is fear and shock. The seasonal energy and time that matches the kidney is winter. Its environmental factor is cold. The color related to kidney energy is black. The taste that goes directly to the kidney is salty. The direction or location is North.

The kidney is the body's energy foundation. It generates the power for the entire body and supports the activities of all other organs. Its main job is to store the concentrated energy-essence, called *Jing*, which transforms into Qi. *Jing* is the "mother" of Qi. It has two components: energy we're born with called Inborn Qi and energy we generate after birth called Acquired Qi. To help my patients understand this concept, I tell them to think of Inborn Qi as an energy "savings account" and Acquired Qi as an energy "checking account." As we've discussed, funds for Acquired Qi are generated by the all-important stomach/spleen partnership. Ideally, your daily life's activities should be supported by your energy checking account. When they're not and

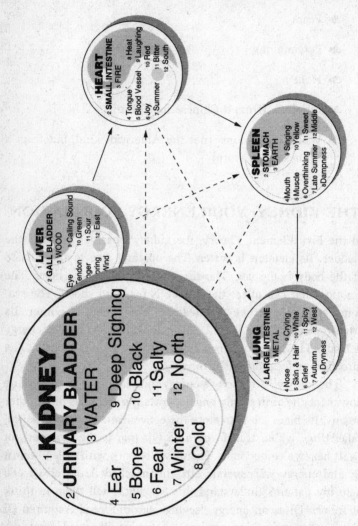

FIVE ELEMENT THEORY

you dip into your energy savings account, you are deficit spending and withdrawing Qi from an irreplaceable asset.

Ancient TCM Tip For Self-Healing

Five foods you can eat to help boost kidney Qi:

- Shellfish: lobster, clams, oysters, shrimp

- Beans: especially black beans

- Bone marrow and bone marrow soup

- Walnuts

- Pine nuts

YOU AND YOUR INBORN QI

Inborn Qi is the portion of your energy foundation inherited from your parents. Its quantity and quality are determined by the quality of your own mother's and father's Qi, the kind of pregnancy your mother had, and the time, place, and nature of your birth. This energy foundation cannot be changed. It's like inheriting land—you may get ten acres or a hundred, it may be rich land or poor. You cannot change your legacy. What is under your control, however, is how you take care of and manage it.

Let's look a little more deeply at Inborn Qi. This energetic force determines your basic constitution, both physical and mental, and governs your growth and development. We know that a house can only be as good as its foundation. How strong and big a "house" you can build for yourself depends on the quality of your energy foundation. The strength of your Inborn Qi also supports your sexual and reproductive functions. Problems such as impotence, infertility, and repetitive miscarriages can indicate a weakness or deficiency in your inherited Qi. The quantity and quality of your Inborn Qi also determines your lifespan. The

Nei Jing says: "Men are born on the earth, but life itself (spirit) is held in the hands of heaven. When the Qi of heaven and earth harmonize, it is called a human being." That's why TCM believes that your lifespan is determined by fate and cannot be changed; how you manage the time and the health heaven has given you is up to you. There are many roads you can choose. You can suffer from stress, unhappiness, and illness all the way, or you can make your journey a peaceful healthy one. It's up to you. The first way uses up Inborn Qi faster than the second. The destination is the same for everyone.

Inborn Qi also relates to genetic problems. When women reach the age of menopause, the overall energy foundation of their "house" begins to weaken. As kidney Qi declines naturally with age, they become more susceptible to whatever genetic flaws they've inherited. The decline of the body's Qi means there is not enough power or strength to control a negative genetic pattern like breast or other cancers that have lived dormant in the body for years. What was contained or kept under control, now can unleash itself. During this time, if the body's organs are already suffering from a dysfunction, or if Qi has stagnated in the meridians over time, then conditions that cause breast cancer can develop. Whichever meridian has the most stagnated Qi becomes the location where a woman is most vulnerable to breast cancer.

KIDNEY ENERGY AND WOMEN

In women, kidney Qi waxes and wanes in seven-year cycles. At the end of the first seven years, a young girl's kidney Qi begins to support her body. You can see this in hair growth and permanent teeth. At fourteen years, this energy reaches its peak, causing the onset of puberty and the beginning of menstruation. A woman in good health flourishes throughout her fertile years, and then around age thirty-five her Qi begins to decline natu-

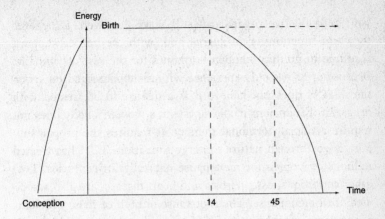

rally. At this point, how quickly it declines is directly related to the way she has taken care of herself and the condition of her Inborn Qi.

Menopause usually occurs between the sixth and seventh cycles, the ages of forty-two and forty-nine. This too is a natural transition and not a medical condition. At this time, kidney Qi begins to drop significantly, menstruation ceases, and signs and symptoms of age may begin to show up (see Diagram). If you take care of yourself well, you can maintain your Inborn Qi, or vital energy, at a higher level for a longer time, delaying menopause and increasing both the length and quality of your life.

In addition to the kidney, women are fortunate enough to possess a second power source that generates Qi—the uterus and ovaries. These organs comprise a special "engine" able to receive, store, and accumulate Qi. Your menstrual cycle lets you accumulate both Qi and blood. It also gives you a special connection between internal and external energies (for example, many women relate to the full moon and it energies), as well as the means to strengthen your body's overall Qi every month. Your uterus and ovaries are also the engines that produce hormones throughout your childbearing years.

TCM believes that even after menopause, if you are healthy,

your reproductive organs can still serve you well. It believes they can function as an engine and, with the proper support, continue to produce enough hormones for the rest of your life. Because of its age-old experience with menopause and its symptoms, TCM does not believe it is a disease to be treated with drugs. In this ancient medical system, a woman's body does not require artificial hormonal therapy. It requires the proper support to go through nature's energy transition. TCM has treated millions of women for menopause naturally for centuries. Two other conditions, osteoporosis and heart disease, are also associated with menopause. The root cause of both of these problems is the same. According to TCM, they spring from a kidney Qi deficiency. TCM has a number of time-tested, natural ways to treat all these conditions.

TCM believes it is essential to understand the importance of your special "engine." If at all possible, TCM recommends against removing the uterus or ovaries. Your uterus is especially vital, because it controls the production of hormones. If you've had a hysterectomy, you're likely to have even more problems going through menopause. If you suffer from menstrual problems such as excessive bleeding and the cause is a Qi deficiency and not tumors or cancer, classical Chinese herbs can offer excellent treatment benefits and can help relieve this problem. Often, just three to five days of herbal therapy can be enough to stop the bleeding. Even after menopause, the reproductive organs still have Qi; they still retain their message, and TCM believes they still have an important purpose. If possible, try to retain these special organs.

Let's return to kidney Qi. There are a number of signs that indicate your kidney Qi is weakening. You may feel cold all the time, a cold that comes from the inside. You may lose your hair, or your sex drive, common problems that come with age. According to TCM, the ears are the "opening" of the kidney and are sustained by its energy. With weak kidney function, your ears may ring; you may suffer from earaches or start to lose your hearing. The kidney is also associated with the bones. As your kidney Qi declines, watch out for your bones—they may become brittle and weak with age. TCM calls the teeth "the surplus of the bone." If you experience problems with your teeth or they start to fall out, you are seeing the effects of kidney Qi deficiency. And one of the most common symptoms related to deficient kidney Qi is lower back pain. Why? The lower back houses the kidney. If your foundation is shaky, how can your house be strong? Some women may experience some of these symptoms well before menopause because, as we've said, kidney Qi often begins to decline around age thirty-five. This is especially true of women who've lived a high-stress life and overdrawn their kidney Qi.

PROTECTING YOUR ENERGY "SAVINGS ACCOUNT"

Most people draw on their savings account of Inborn Qi without knowing or thinking. Often, we use these precious energy funds wastefully. As we've seen, TCM theory states that when this account is used up, it's time to die. So there is every reason to conserve Inborn Qi. Conservation, if we follow the way of nature, is the most important principle relating to the kidney, where your energy "savings account" is stored. Your kidney corresponds with the winter season. Think of what happens during the winter: trees lose their leaves, animals hibernate, birds fly south, lakes and ponds freeze over. Nature withdraws into herself; she conserves her energy and she rests.

In the same way, you should recognize the value of your unique energy foundation and do everything possible to conserve it. The *Nei Jing* says, "The sage knows that *Jing*/Essence is the most precious substance in the body. Like the root of a tree, it should be protected and hidden from 'thieves'." What are these Qi-robbing thieves? Stress and overwork are certainly two. One of the biggest "thieves," in terms of kidney Qi, is sex. Sexual activity draws heavily on the energy of your kidney. It makes your heart beat faster; it makes your whole body function at an accelerated rate, which causes large expenditures of Qi. During breast cancer treatment, I recommend that my patients have sex in moderation so that they can conserve more Qi for self-healing. Overall, TCM advises moderation in sex—especially for older people, or those with a weak energy foundation.

TCM principles state that it is impossible to add to kidney Qi, or your energy "savings account." But even if this kidney Qi cannot be increased, you can slow its decline. There are many simple ways to do this. Resting and conserving energy is one. Qigong practice is another. Qigong is the ancient self-healing energy system that can help get your body back in balance and bring it up to its maximum function. This eliminates Qi wasted through dysfunction in the organs or the disruption of healthy partnerships among your organs. Qigong can also help your body function more efficiently, which reduces the amount of Qi it needs to function daily. And, if your body is balanced, your spleen and stomach will be able to extract more energy from the foods you eat, thereby further reducing the demand for more kidney Qi. The best time to strengthen your kidney Qi with Qigong is before any problems arise. As the ancient Chinese say: "You should dig the well before you get thirsty." The most important part of this book is the *Wu Ming* Meridian Therapy in Chapter 16. Incorporate these movements into your daily life and you will be amazed at the healing benefits you'll receive.

Here's an example of how Qigong can help save Qi. Before we go further, remember that Qi, of course, is intangible, formless and unmeasurable. The effect of Qi, however, can be observed. If you have strong Qi, then you are healthy. All healthy people have strong Qi. Now, let's suppose like so many people you have some health problems. You need one hundred units of Qi every day for your body to function well. In this theoretical amount, though, at least 30 to 40 percent of it is wasted in dealing with healing physical problems and addressing internal communications issues between organs. Ideally, these hundred units of Qi should be withdrawn from your checking account, which comes from your spleen and stomach. But, suppose you can only produce seventy units from these two organs. Your savings account of kidney Qi must make up the rest. The Qi must come from one of these two systems; that is the natural law of how the body operates You can easily see that poor digestive function is another thief, stealing your kidney's special, but finite, treasure.

Most of us routinely withdraw funds from our "savings account" of kidney Qi for daily expenditures, when we should be relying on our "checking account" of Qi produced by our spleen/stomach. It is difficult to overemphasize the importance of drawing from your Acquired Qi. Qigong practice can help you fix your body's health problems, make the communications among your organ systems much more efficient, and improve the quality and quantity of these energy transfers. It can actually help you use less Qi, look younger and feel healthier. Best of all, it can save you that 30 to 40 percent of wasted Qi, which can help you tremendously if you have breast cancer or want to prevent its recurrence.

I like to joke with my patients when they ask me "How can I stop withdrawing Qi from my savings account?" I tell them for thousands of years, many, many emperors, empresses, Taoist masters, and humble workers have tried to answer this question. If they could have, then they would have lived forever in a youthful condition. In theory because we are part of nature, and nature regenerates itself, we should be able to do this. Sorry to say, but the reality is that every day we draw a little bit of our kidney Qi. And, every day we grow a little older. So, you can observe the use of your own savings account. Each gray hair, each wrinkle, each tooth gone, hearing loss, worsening vision, all indicate that you are depleting this irreplaceable asset.

THE DAILY MIRACLE OF ACQUIRED QI

As I've said, Inborn Qi cannot be changed; luckily Acquired Qi can. If you're smart, you'll add to your energy "checking account" daily. Eat good quality food and learn how to conserve and manage your Qi. For example: go to bed at a reasonable hour so you don't use up Qi to remain awake. Don't eat too late so that your body has to spend extra Qi all night long to digest your food, when it should be at rest. When cold weather comes, dress adequately so that your body doesn't have to spend extra Qi to keep you warm. You're probably thinking that you've heard these things before, right? Maybe your mother said these things to you. Their true purpose is to save Qi. Acquired Qi supports the function of all your organs and helps maintain your body's ability to regulate and heal itself. Through your creation and management of Acquired Qi, you have the chance to experience a daily miracle that will help strengthen the power and harmonious functioning of your body. This gives hope for many because there is always the power and potential to be 100 percent the best for your body's individual system, whatever its limitations. Understanding how to nurture and increase Qi also puts the power of healing in your own hands. You are a unique holistic system—a combination of genetic gifts and daily Qi accumulation. How you take care of this system is of the utmost importance to the prevention or control of breast cancer. Chapter 17 offers a wealth of ancient knowledge to help you strengthen your energy "checking account."

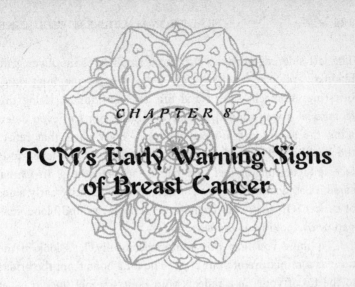

CHAPTER 8
TCM's Early Warning Signs of Breast Cancer

YOUR body continually sends you messages about how it feels and how well it's functioning. Understanding these messages could save your life. The following body signals are based on the TCM theory that the body is a microcosm of the greater Universe—"As above, so below." TCM practitioners believe that the macrocosm always contains the microcosm. The universe is reflected in our bodies; the condition of the body is reflected in the condition of its parts, and vice versa. This TCM principle helps practitioners to identify internal problems by analyzing exterior signs. Two often-used diagnostic tools are readings of the tongue and the pulse. For instance, if you walked into my office I would be able to tell if you had a digestive system problem by the color of your tongue. Your tongue's shape would also have meaning to me. Large, teethlike marks on the tongue's edge would indicate to me that your body is suffering from an overall Qi deficiency. Individuals with chronic fatigue syndrome, or those who are undergoing chemotherapy, often exhibit this sign.

With pulse diagnoses, the practitioner can feel subtle vibrations in each wrist area that reflect the Qi of different organs.

The left side encompasses the heart, small intestine, liver, gall-bladder, and bladder. The right side includes the lung, large intestine, stomach, spleen and life gate, or kidney. Using this technique, a well-trained, sensitive TCM doctor can even determine the sex of a two-week-old fetus. Body parts that reflect the health of the whole body also include your ear, eye, nose, face, and bottom of feet and palms, among others. In China, some TCM doctors still use ear diagnosis to identify early signs of cancer. Or, they can diagnose Qi deficiencies and blood stagnation by looking at the eyes.

To show you how this works specifically, let's look at the nose as a miniature of your body. The long bone from the bridge to the tip of your nose reflects your body's spine; the curves at the nostrils reflect the health of your hip joints. The middle of the tip of your nose reflects the condition of your stomach. If you have skin problems on your nose, I am able to recognize which organs are causing them. A red nose means that the stomach is suffering from a condition of excess heat. This principle applies to almost all the body parts. Each one represents the entire body in miniature. Reflexology is based on this principle. For example, the bottom of your foot is regarded as a map of your entire body. Your hand is also a body map. So are your face, your tongue, your nose and the bone of your index finger, and so on.

Following is a list of external signs that TCM uses to evaluate the condition of your internal Qi or life force, and how a specific organ is doing. You can use this information to check yourself from time to time and to identify problems in the making. This will give you the knowledge and the information to help prevent various health conditions from worsening. If you have any of the following symptoms, don't ignore them. I recommend that you try and fix them as soon as possible.

Taste: Do you experience any of the following tastes on a regular basis?

- Bitter: Your body's organs are suffering from excess internal heat.
- Sweet: Your stomach and spleen have excess heat.
- Salty: Your kidney has excess heat.
- Sour: Your liver cannot work in harmony with your stomach and spleen.

Tongue

- Purple color on the sides: Your liver energy or blood has stagnation.
- Teeth-like marks on the side: Your digestive system is weak; you are suffering from an overall Qi deficiency. This is seen particularly during or after chemotherapy and radiation.
- Dark red with deep lines or fissures: Your body is loosing tremendous energy. This is seen particularly after radiation and chemotherapy.
- Thick white coating: Your stomach has poor digestion.
- Thick yellow coating: Your stomach has tremendous heat.
- Purple or greenish coating: A serious sign that could indicate lung cancer.
- Blisters under the tongue: If they turn purple or dark in color, you have a serious sign that a tumor or cancer might develop somewhere in your body. Be careful.

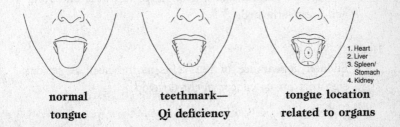

normal tongue

teethmark— Qi deficiency

tongue location related to organs

1. Heart
2. Liver
3. Spleen/ Stomach
4. Kidney

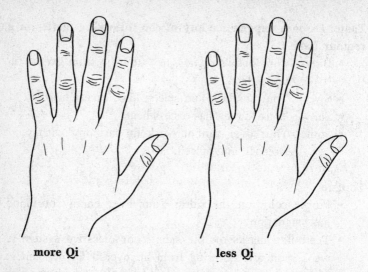

more Qi   **less Qi**

Nails

- Thumb, middle, and index fingers have straight black lines: Your digestive system or reproductive system may get cancer.
- Easily broken nails or nails that are not smooth or shiny: Your liver function is sluggish or poor.
- Half moons with little or no white areas: Your liver Qi is deficient. The less white space that shows, the more acute the Qi or energy deficiency.

Teeth

- Bleeding gums: Your body's overall Qi is low.
- Swollen or painful gums: Your large intestine and stomach are overheated.

Heel

- Sudden appearance of red veins at the heel: A serious sign that breast cancer might develop.

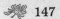

DREAMS

For thousands of years, TCM practitioners have used dreams as an important tool to diagnose and treat disease. Be especially careful if you continually have nightmares where you are fighting for something and never win; where you are running from something, but never escape; where you're hiding from something, but are always caught. If you already have cancer, these nightmares are internal energy messages telling you that your condition is about to worsen. On the other hand, if you always dream that you are happy and successful, or go through a door with sunshine on the other side, or you drive through a beautiful forest and the sun breaks through, or a bridge connects you to another area, your problem is starting to improve.

If you always dream that you are traveling, or taking any kind of transportation such as a train or plane or even an elevator but you never reach your destination, this means your body is warning you of a serious Qi stagnation somewhere inside. There is usually a related dream that can indicate the location of this stagnation. For instance, you might dream that someone gives you a flower that you pin over your chest. Or, a meeting badge might prick you in the chest area; or an insect like a bee or an animal like a snake might appear and sting or bite you in this area—be careful. TCM understands these as signs of serious Qi stagnation problems leading to breast cancer.

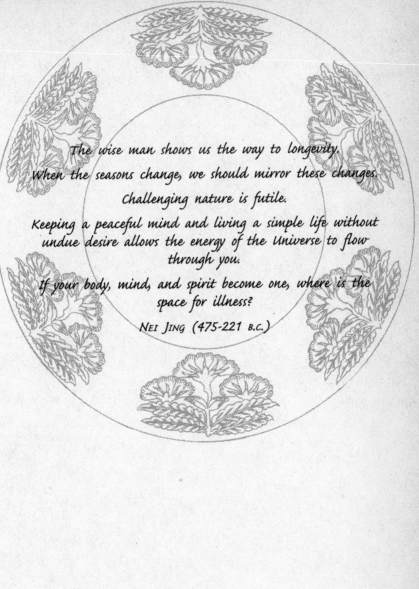

The wise man shows us the way to longevity.

When the seasons change, we should mirror these changes.

Challenging nature is futile.

Keeping a peaceful mind and living a simple life without undue desire allows the energy of the Universe to flow through you.

If your body, mind, and spirit become one, where is the space for illness?

Nei Jing (475–221 b.c.)

CHAPTER 9

TCM: Treating the Source Not the Symptoms

LET'S look at disease or illness the way TCM sees them. First, it regards the presenting symptom (your migraine headache, for example) as a signal from the body of a deeper situation that is affecting either an organ or a meridian (or both) that must be addressed. Rather than naming the condition, TCM diagnoses it in terms of either an energy function disorder or a Qi imbalance, as these states relate to the particular organ or organs that are distressed. TCM sees this symptom as being unique to your own special energy pattern. In other words, your migraine headache is not the same as your girlfriend's, or your mother's, or your colleague's, even if they share all the same characteristics. Why? Quite simply because you are not they and they are not you. In fact, TCM understands that six meridians run up through the head. Any one or a combination of them can cause your headache. So, TCM recognizes that there are 720 different possible causes of headaches ($6 \times 5 \times 4 \times 3 \times 2 \times 1 = 720$). Looking at it this way, you can begin to understand why the medication that your friend recommends as the "fastest working" one she's ever taken does nothing for you.

From the TCM standpoint, everything about you is unique.

Each of you is an individual and TCM focuses its attention on your own individual problem-producing dynamics. By treating you as an individual, TCM can treat your migraine effectively. How? It can get to the root cause of it. If you have a health problem, your body is out of balance and offers the ideal environment within which unbalanced energy can comfortably exist. Without the right kind of help to rebalance your organ system, this condition is unlikely to leave you on its own. The real healer helps create the opportunity for the patient to change her energy field and reconnect to her state of internal harmony. Reaching this means reaching the root cause of her problem. If she can do this, then the disease or illness can be healed.

TCM TREATMENT PRINCIPLES

❧ Treat the root cause.

❧ Strengthen the body's immune system.

❧ Harmonize the function of the body's organs.

❧ Adapt treatment to the specific needs of the individual: "who you are" (body type, genetics), "where you are" (geographical location), "how you are" (physical condition and lifestyle) and "when you are" (age, time of day and season, time of symptom).

The various treatments discussed in this chapter must be applied using the above principles. How does TCM approach treatment? First, as we've seen, it takes a highly individualistic approach. The TCM practitioner is trained to understand that effective treatment depends on: where you are; when you are; how you are; and who you are. In other words, location, time (of day or season), your current condition and genetic blueprint are all specific factors that determine the course (and the outcome) of your treatment. A good TCM doctor combines two objectives in the selection of treatments: he or she will first try to address the root cause. At the same time, he or she will also try to prevent the problem from going deeper and affecting other organs. The first step in this process is to determine whether the symptoms indicate an emergency or whether they represent some sort of chronic condition. TCM treatments generally include herbal therapy, acupuncture, Chinese medical massage, known as Tuina, or acupressure, Qigong, the skillful prescription of foods, and the application of ancient psychology. Above all, TCM recognizes the body's capacity to heal itself and works at nurturing this ability.

I'm often asked if certain conditions respond better to TCM than Western medicine. There are many that do. TCM is good for strengthening the immune system and for treating chronic conditions such as lupus, chronic stomachaches or headaches, chronic fatigue syndrome, allergies, asthma, skin problems, hypoglycemia, to name a few. These kinds of internal problems take time and patience to treat and to gain maximum results. For conditions like tennis elbow, sprains, stiff necks and muscle pulls, TCM is often faster and more effective than Western treatment, especially because there are no side effects.

Many patients who come to me are pretty much at the end of their ropes. As you've seen from the examples in this book, a number of these individuals have tried many things to rid themselves of their health problem. Some have spent small fortunes and gone for longer than a decade in search of relief. Often I see a patient who has undergone a battery of Western medical tests and who has been told that she is "fine." The patient, however, is acutely aware that she is not fine (nor is she crazy, as some of my patients have been told). Some of these women suffer from a function disorder—one or more of their organ systems is not working properly. Others may have an added physical problem like a non-cancerous tumor. Often dramatic changes can occur in relatively brief treatment periods if we communicate well and work together productively. I think some of the case histories outlined here give you a good idea of why and how this can happen. These changes are not the result of "quick fixes"; they are routinely permanent reversals of conditions that have been addressed by finally treating the source and not the symptoms.

My first-time patients are often unaware of what to expect from a visit to a TCM doctor. In my practice, my first order of business is to explain to them that I am a classically trained doctor of TCM. I am not a Western medical doctor with some TCM training. My classical training lies rooted in the tradition of the best ancient doctors. These individuals were, above all, expected to be Qigong or energy masters and deeply versed in the understanding of Qi. They were also expected to be expert martial artists, since the martial arts are intended for healing first and self-defense second. Another skill required of them was the ability to make up ancient herbal formulas in the TCM apothecary and, when needed, adapt them to the specific needs of each patient. They were also taught how to apply TCM's fundamental principles and theories to their patients' conditions. Without this kind of training and experience with Qi, it is still possible to practice the techniques of TCM, but not its true spirit and power. Many of these ancient doctors were also passed information from their masters.

The real secret behind TCM is Qi. No matter which technique is used, be it herbs, or acupressure, or acupuncture, etc., the real secret behind these treatments is always Qi. The challenge is for the energy practitioner to spark the patient's own Qi to respond. You can compare this with a car that needs a jump start because its battery has died. If the battery is in good shape, a good charge will make it work again. My own master, professor Xi-hua Xu, always reminds me that a really good energy healer begins first by creating an energy bond between the doctor and the patient. Without this energy or Qi connection, no matter how good a doctor, the treatment process can only take place at the symptom level. But, with a strong energy bond, the healer and patient can actually amplify their energy field exponentially, to help the person's own healing power overcome the disease or illness. Because TCM views the treatment modality as a partnership, it is vital that both partners get to know each other. It is the whole person, not the disease, that requires attention—her body, mind, and spirit—if good results are to be gained. Therefore, all psychological issues bear on ultimate treatment success. Spending quality time with the patient is an essential part of the treatment. You can begin to appreciate the difference between the TCM and Western approach to disease and healing.

Because Western society causes so many stress-related conditions, the skilled TCM practitioner spends a lot of time helping the patient realize that her unbalanced emotional reactions to situations are what is really behind the physical problems. As TCM says: "Your heart can create heaven or hell." To put it into more modern terms: "It's not what happens to you, but how you take it." For TCM, emotional/psychological factors are crucial parts of the puzzle; without this understanding and the context of the yin and yang and Five Element theories, treatment is incomplete.

It is helpful to a new patient to describe what she can expect in the upcoming appointment. I tell her the TCM examination is made up of four diagnostic methods: looking (facial color, shape, eye and tongue color, emotional state); smell and hearing (body and mouth odor, noise from chest and nose); asking (talking about the patient's problem—especially probing for clues that relate to frequency, time of day, degree, type), and touch (pulse diagnosis). I try to educate the patient that good TCM doctors are trained to understand that many physical problems are connected with emotional issues, which, in turn, are the root of the major presenting condition. It is very important for me as a TCM practitioner to understand how my patient "feels" and what kind of emotional or spiritual issues are affecting her life. This is especially critical with breast cancer patients. I spend a lot of time with a patient who has breast problems or breast cancer. I want to show them how the stresses they accept and deal with daily damage the way their body functions. I try to teach her that, from the exact location of her breast cancer, we can identify which of her organs or meridians is being affected by stress or other emotional problems.

CHOOSING A DOCTOR OF TCM

It is not surprising that the use of alternative (I like to think of it as complementary) medicine, as it is called, is growing rapidly in the West. A 1998 study in the *Journal of the American Medical Association* shows that alternative therapies are being used by four out of every ten Americans. The study also shows that $27 billion dollars was spent on remedies ranging from herbal pills to acupuncture. It's interesting to note that most of these dollars are coming out of the consumer's own pocket. With so many people searching for answers to their health needs, it is important to know how to select quality care. This is very important when choosing a practitioner of TCM.

When a patient moves, I am often asked how to find a TCM doctor. The truth is, it isn't easy. It is not like selecting a Western physician. When choosing a TCM practitioner, I tell them to trust their intuition. If the treatment isn't working within a short time, I tell her that she must talk things over with her TCM doctor to uncover why. If she does not feel that she can establish a trusting working partnership, if she observes that the doctor cannot skillfully apply the TCM principles discussed above, then I advise her to find another doctor. Otherwise, I tell her "You are being treated in a Western way—substituting acupuncture needles for drugs, and substituting technique for theory. Your symptoms may be receiving treatment, but the source is still being ignored." It is my responsibility to point out a very real danger in this situation. If the practitioner does not have a deep understanding of TCM principles and theories, he or she can do a lot of harm to the patient. Why? It's because they are dealing with the body's natural healing Qi and by misdirecting it can cause more internal problems than when the patient started. The patient herself, though, may never connect her future health problems to this set of circumstances.

There are several ways you can identify whether or not a TCM practitioner has the appropriate kind of training and insight to help you. For your own education, take the time to read over the main principles and theories of TCM in Chapters 5 and 6. These have remained unchanged for many thousands of years. Also review the Five Element Theory so you can become familiar with the relationships among the five major organ pairs and the internal and external factors that influence their healthy function and balance. Try to see where your physical discomfort fits. What organs might it be related to? Which emotions may be playing a role in your problem?

Now when you select a TCM practitioner, you have some common ground. When you meet, does the TCM practitioner use the classical four-stage diagnosis methodology outlined above? Second, does he or she take the time to create that indispensable energy bond with you, or do you get a ten-minute work-up and then get sent to a room for acupuncture treatment? (Remember it's the energy relationship that heals, the energy vehicle of the needles or herbs are of secondary importance.) Does he or she help you realize there are daily lifestyle choices that must change in order to heal? If you have no benefit after a few treatments, does he or she sit with you to redesign treatment to get at the problem another way? When you discuss your symptoms, can he or she work with you to identify factors that are causing them? For example, do they understand that your breast tenderness, PMS, and menstrual cramps are all related to a stressed lifestyle and a liver function disorder? Do they understand that your migraine headache that occurs each day at 8:00 A.M. means that your stomach's energy is not functioning properly? When searching for a TCM doctor (or acupuncturist or herbalist), I believe your best choice is one who understands and practices TCM in accordance with its ancient principles and theories.

TCM TREATMENTS

As we've seen, the TCM practitioner's role is simple and complex at the same time. His or her job is to balance the opposing, yet complementary yin and yang energies within the patient and strengthen her own healing ability so she can heal herself. A variety of vehicles are used for this purpose: foods for healing, herbal therapy, acupuncture, acupressure, moxibustion (the application of heated herbs to a particular acupoint or meridian), Qigong, the ancient self-healing energy practice, and Chinese psychology.

Food

TCM has a long history of using food as medicine. Ancient doctors understood, from an energy perspective, which foods could heal which organs. This information has been passed down and been in use for thousands of years. In Chapter 17, I have compiled a selective list of healing foods and classical herbs, as well as descriptions of how to use them. This is accompanied by healing recipes using these ingredients, which can help many women. They are useful if you are dealing with the side effects of breast cancer treatment, as well as if you want to strengthen your body to prevent breast cancer. You can also use this information in conjunction with your understanding of various symptoms to help heal certain early stage conditions so that they do not progress to more serious health problems. To the best of my knowledge, this comprehensive healing resource has never been presented to Western audiences like this before.

Foods are natural elements and, when used properly, produce virtually no side effects. Eating good quality foods for healing is something you can do every single day to help yourself. TCM has a unique understanding of foods as medicine that goes beyond the physical properties of nutrition, calories, or vitamins. TCM has mapped out the healing energies and essences of specific foods and the organs they go to. Remember that we discussed that food comes into the body and turns into essence via the spleen/stomach partnership; this nutritive essence is sent up to the lung where it receives its instructions about where to go. The lung, in turn, knows that each food is coded with its own essence and understanding of which organ it should go to. Let's see what happens when you make a delicious soup with black beans, sweet potatoes, scallions, ginger, and cinnamon. After the stomach digests this food, the spleen will send the nutritive essence of each one to the lung. Then, the lung will transform these essences into Qi and distribute the Qi to specific organs. The Qi of the black beans and cinnamon will go immediately to your kidney; the Qi or essence of the sweet potato and ginger will enter your stomach and spleen; the scallion's Qi will go directly to your liver. Each of these foods will enhance or strengthen the organ they relate to. This energy blueprint is even more important than the foods' physical properties.

Today, there is a lot of ongoing research in the West as scientists attempt to prove conclusively that certain foods, like broccoli, carrots, kale, etc., can help prevent or heal breast cancer. Until science can go beyond the physical properties of things and apply the concept of energy, how these foods benefit breast cancer patients might remain a mystery. Well-trained TCM doctors know how to create various food recipes for healing purposes. (See Chapter 17 for more information and healing recipes you can use to address certain symptoms that are early warning signs of breast cancer.)

TCM Herbs

Today, many consumers try to help themselves when they're sick. This is especially true if they have a chronic condition that Western medicine cannot cure. Another group of consumers wants to prevent disease or illness. Both groups frequently turn to natural food supplements, vitamins, tonics, herbal compounds, etc. You name the problem, whether it is osteoporosis, heart disease, brain function improvement, there is something on the market you can take that supposedly helps. I always tell my patients to think about this concept carefully: "You have a symptom; you take a pill for it." In the case of single herbs or herbal formulas, the only difference is that they are replacing chemical substances with natural compounds. They are still not treating the root cause. Too often, I see patients ingesting large quantities of these pills, vitamins, tonics, and many other things. I ask them how they know if these things will help them? How do they know that these substances won't harm them? Most laboratories haven't tested this kind of real-life usage (or abuse, in some cases), nor have they tested their products in these vast combinations. I also tell my patients to think twice before ingesting large quantities of these substances because they all must pass through the stomach, the liver, and the kidney.

A vast apothecary of herbs is available to TCM practitioners for healing purposes. In the East, the concept of "herb" has a broader meaning than in the West. An herb can mean any natural material used in a formula. Ancient TCM doctors were skilled at using all kinds of things for healing. Stones, bones, dirt, glass, wood, bark, leaves, roots, petals, stems, and just about every conceivable animal part could be included in an herbal recipe.

Classical herbal remedies are based on a particular combination of selected herbs; the result is a unique medicine that is stronger than the sum of its parts. One way to understand this concept is to regard the TCM herbal ingredient as a football player—not a tennis player. In a TCM formulation, the team is what counts. Every herb has a specific job: some herbs are used to directly impact a given condition; some are used to help tune up certain organs; some help strengthen an organ's Qi or power; some are used to flush out toxic material; others block the disease from becoming worse—anticipating its next move—and some herbs help create an inhospitable internal environment where the disease or toxic invader is no longer comfortable.

This last technique is very interesting. Let me describe one approach TCM uses for attacking some medical conditions. Imagine a fish tank with a large enemy fish you wish to destroy. One way to do this would be to analyze the fish, check its speed, size, habits, and the like. Then you would prepare a bullet and shoot the fish. Sometimes you might hit the mark; sometimes not. TCM takes a different approach. Basically, it would add something to the fish's water that would gradually change the entire environment, which, in turn, would control the fish, cause it to perform differently, or cause it die.

To illustrate the TCM concept of living "with" a particular condition or situation, consider the following examples. There is one famous classical herbal formulation for parasites that is many centuries old. This formulation controls the parasite by putting it to sleep rather than killing it. While the parasite still lives within the body, it has been rendered harmless. TCM believes you can live with a wide variety of conditions, as long as they don't bother you. Let's look at another example—gallstones. Ancient herbal formulations were used to alter the body's internal Qi and environment so that the gallstone symptoms could be eliminated (not suppressed). Although the patient might experience some occasional mild pain, he or she would benefit tremendously from saving the organ itself. Why is the gallbladder so significant? The *Nei Jing* considers it an indispensable organ because it can coordinate and influence the function of all eleven other organs. Its meridian is the only one that makes a connection with the other eleven as well. It is also the seat of decision making. Because of the nature of the gallbladder's function, a missing one may eventually lead to Alzheimer's disease.

A knowledgeable, classically trained TCM doctor will formulate his herbal remedies to accomplish at least three things: help relieve or control the condition's symptoms; address the root cause of the condition as diagnosed; and deliver the right combination of herbs to protect and strengthen the organ(s) that the condition may affect next. A good TCM doctor will never use herbs to cover up or suppress symptoms.

Combining TCM herbs is an art form that cannot be learned from a medical textbook. Here is another important principle that will help you understand that combining many herbs in one formula (like ginseng, *Gingko biloba,* black cohosh) may, at best, only give you the benefits of each individual herb. The effect is not always additive, in fact, because the combination is not based on comprehensive herbal theory, it has the potential to cause problems. When I explain this concept to my patients, I tell them: consider how many times Hollywood combines a famous director and a beautiful movie star; just putting them together is no guarantee of a box office hit! Or, look at the world of computers. It would be nice if a PC worked with a MAC, but even if they're made compatible, you can still experience problems. Much of the inspired knowledge about TCM herbal formulations has been passed from master to student over many generations. During my lifetime, I have been privileged to receive this kind of knowledge from several extraordinary masters. Again, herbal treatments are energy treatments. It is the essence or Qi, not the scientific properties that heal.

Acupuncture and Moxibustion

Acupuncture and moxibustion are based on meridian theories. The meridians, as we have seen, are energy pathways that form a network throughout the entire body. Needles or heat (in the case of moxibustion) are used to relieve an energy blockage at certain key acupoints to help the body's Qi flow smoothly. They also can be used to readjust an organ's function to achieve harmony inside the body. Some health conditions respond very well to acupuncture; some respond to moxibustion. Some conditions do not respond to either—or even both, when used complementarily. Again, the well-trained TCM doctor will know when and how to apply each of these specific treatments.

Sometimes, people say that acupuncture has not helped them. This doesn't mean that acupuncture doesn't work. Acupuncture might not be appropriate for their condition. Their acupuncturist may not be skillful enough to treat their problem, or the acupuncturist's energy cannot match with their own energy. For example, pain can come from two causes: external forces like sports injury or car accidents, among other things. Or, pain can come from an internal Qi deficiency or Qi stagnation, like migraine or allergy headaches, menstrual cramps, chronic lower back or neck pain. Because the cause of each of these conditions is different, the treatment should be different. External pain conditions are fairly easy to treat and usually produce benefits quickly. Internal conditions of pain are actually quite complicated and require more knowledge to treat. This is because, unless the root cause is identified, the practitioner may only succeed in relieving symptoms and the risk of pain recurring remains.

As an example, I have a patient who has had lower back pain for years. When we first met she told me that she had been to many acupuncturists. A friend of hers referred her to me because of our successful relationship in treating her lower back pain in a very short time. This woman related how the first few acupuncture treatments with several practitioners had usually relieved her pain, but then it would return. When I asked her how these acupuncturists had diagnosed her, she said that no one had done a four-part diagnosis. No one had asked her about herself and her emotions and her lifestyle habits. Nor did these practitioners spend very much time with her. They put her in a room with acupuncture needles in the location of her pain for thirty minutes, then sent her on her way. She would feel some relief after these treatments, which gave her hope that acupuncture could eventually cure this problem. But always the pain returned within one or two days, sometimes even the same day. During our first appointment, I told her that I would do my best to help her, but that she needed to realize that just because I was able to help her friend's lower back pain, did not necessarily mean that I could help hers. Her friend's lower back pain was caused by a car accident. Because she had no external injury, I told her I believed her chronic back pain pointed to an internal cause.

During my diagnosis, I found that her pain was related to a kidney Qi deficiency. I could also tell that she had liver Qi stagnation. Some of her symptoms included the fact that her whole body always felt cold; she also had urinary frequency. Her lower back pain was particularly acute during her menstrual cycle. She also suffered from cramps during her menstrual cycle. All these symptoms helped me recognize the source of her problem. Within four treatments, she told me she had about 80 percent ongoing relief from pain. I advised her that complete healing would come from strengthening her kidney Qi and that she needed to conserve her energy for healing by eating foods to boost her kidney Qi and resting.

Highly trained TCM doctors practice energy acupuncture

that, again, is a technique that cannot be learned from medical texts. Energy acupuncture includes deep insight into what has caused the health problem, as well as into what organs and areas are affected. As we've seen with the above story, putting needles where there is pain without proper and deep diagnosis may create some benefits. But, this is not the true, powerful TCM acupuncture of the ancients. In the end, acupuncture is simply a communications vehicle between the doctor's Qi and patient's Qi. It is the knowledge, skill and energy level of the doctor that makes the acupuncture work, not just the needles or the acupoints.

Even though acupuncture has been in use to treat pain and many other conditions in China for several thousands of years, it only became known in the United States in the early 1970s. Today, the Food and Drug Administration (FDA) estimates that more than $500 million a year is spent on treatments involving acupuncture and that Americans are now making between nine and twelve million visits annually to practitioners. One very positive advance for acupuncture therapy in the United States was its acceptance by the National Institutes of Health (NIH) in November 1997 as an effective treatment for postoperative dental pain, nausea and vomiting caused by anesthesia, chemotherapy, or pregnancy. In China, TCM practioners use acupuncture to treat a far broader range of health conditions.

Moxibustion

As described earlier, moxibustion uses a stick of compressed herbal material that is lit and used for applying heat over a specific meridian or to a specific acupoint to relieve a Qi blockage or generate vital energy. Moxibustion is particularly good for breast cancer treatment because of its ability to help dispel the cold yin energy of cancer and generate additional Qi. (See Chapter 18 and learn about the secret energy healing gates you can massage.) As with acupuncture, moxibustion should be practiced with the same deep understanding. Generally speaking, any kind of symptoms relating to or caused by excess cold, like the common cold, or conditions of internal cold like menstrual cramps, or bed wetting can be helped by moxibustion.

Acupressure

Classical TCM acupressure is called *Tuina*. It is the use of special hand techniques or tools to stimulate meridians or acupoints. Though the techniques are different, acupressure is as effective as acupuncture. For some conditions, acupressure is more useful and easier on the patient. For example, sports injuries like tennis elbow or simple sprains respond better to acupressure. Sometimes acupressure and acupuncture together can accelerate healing benefits. *Tuina* requires more physical strength, more study, more training, and more technical skill than acupuncture. In China, in universities of TCM, there are separate majors—one for acupuncture, one for acupressure. Even in TCM hospitals, a patient can be directed to two separate departments for treatment. Acupressure is a medical treatment and is not the same as body massage.

Qigong

It is difficult to say how old the practice of Qigong is. Some believe it goes back more than five thousand years. The word Qigong literally means "energy work," but the actual practice is far deeper than its description. Qigong is a self-healing discipline that allows the practitioner to gain control of and direct his or her own life force. Its biggest benefit is that it can develop your intuition and let you see the world in a different way. The view is one that can take you beyond five senses. This self-healing energy system is a unique tool that women with breast cancer can use to improve their health problems; others can use it to help prevent breast cancer.

There are several distinct Qigong traditions: Taoist, Confucian, Buddhist, martial arts, and medical. It is this last form of Qigong that is beginning to attract a great deal of attention from Western audiences. I say "beginning" because Qigong was suppressed during the Chinese Cultural Revolution, which lasted roughly from 1965 to 1976. Qigong never died out in practice; around 1978, it began its rise in popularity again in China. Today, it is estimated that more than seventy million Chinese practice some form of Qigong daily. Today, more and more people around the world are becoming interested in this ancient energy practice. In 1988, the Chinese held the first world conference for showcasing Qigong medical research. The conferences have grown steadily over the past decade and been held in Tokyo, Japan, and Berkeley, California.

In China, medical practitioners have found Qigong effective in treating a wide variety of health conditions, including drug abuse and obesity. In hospitals and clinics across China, Qigong is routinely prescribed to treat arthritis, asthma, bowel problems, diabetes, migraines, hypertension, rheumatism, neuralgia, stress, ulcers, and many others. As we have discussed, Qigong has also been used successfully to treat cancers and reduce or even eliminate debilitating side effects of radiation and chemotherapy. It also can bring special relief to those suffering from chronic pain, and other chronic conditions that affect the digestive, respiratory, nervous, and cardiovascular systems.

Qigong practice has been documented to speed recovery from surgery and sports and other kinds of injuries. I have had great success with prescribing Qigong for a number of patients to help them recover more rapidly from devastating injuries, like car accidents.

Some of the amazing things that Qigong can do for an individual are: strengthen the immune system, lower blood pressure, adjust pulse rates, help alter metabolic rates, adjust oxygen demand, harmonize endocrine system functions, regulate some of the body's basic building blocks, and even slow the process of aging. Above all, the Qigong practitioner learns through her own experience that there is no separation between the body, mind, and spirit.

One of the most important benefits of Qigong is this deep integration, which allows you to connect your emotions, mind, body and spirit. It is one of the most powerful prescriptions a TCM doctor can use because it works directly on the body's energy system. Practicing Qigong is a serious undertaking. It can help make your whole life change. It is not uncommon in China for women to recover from breast cancer by practicing Qigong.

As we have seen, literally millions of people in China practice this self-healing energy system. Qigong, however, should not be confused with pure physical exercise. Many studies have been done on Qigong and it is generally acknowledged that in addition to its powers of integration, it offers the benefits of aerobics, meditation, and more. It is an essential prescription for some of my patients and ideally addresses many of their problems. I often teach my patients one or two simple Qigong movements to help them reawaken their healing ability and to speed up their healing process. This is good for them because they now have a tool they can use to heal themselves should the same problem occur again. Qigong is particularly good for healing problems that Western medicine cannot identify; usually these are function problems that do not show up on scientific tests.

In China, there are literally thousands of Qigong systems; some are ancient systems passed along for many generations. Some are "instant systems" created by modern masters. Currently, very few Qigong systems have been seen or taught in the United States. In my center's school in New York, I teach Taoist *Wu Ming* Qigong, which traces its lineage back to the ancient masters Lao Tzu and Chuang Tzu. Each Qigong system works differently: some are easy to learn, but deliver few benefits; some are difficult to learn and the benefits are difficult to achieve; some are difficult to learn, but yield great benefits. I believe the best Qigong system should be easy to learn and should allow you to achieve great benefits.

Generally speaking, Qigong systems fall into two separate categories. The first is based on postures and movements that stimulate your internal energy to help heal yourself. In this case, the practitioner must follow the master's directions precisely to gain any benefits from the system. Results depend on correct posture, how much time you practice, and how well your master can teach. In this system, the connection to posture and getting it correct is more important than the relationship between student and master. With this type of system, the benefits are in proportion to the amount of personal effort you put into the practice.

The second category uses movements and postures, but in a different way. They are used to guide the power of the "energy message" from master to student. Doing the forms or postures correctly is not overly important—they are merely the "the vehicle or transportation" for getting the energy message from master to student. (The concept is similar to using acupuncture needles as a communications vehicle to move energy from the TCM practitioner to the patient. The success of the treatment depends on who uses the needle.) The student then uses this message to help restore and refunction his or her internal Qi.

The first type of Qigong is like having your computer professor teach you how to write a program that can help improve your health. Using his instructions, you must write your own program and then use it by yourself in your personal computer. There are no other connections or instructions. How well you can apply this program now depends on you and your own intuition.

With the second type of Qigong, the professor first reveals to you the principles and theories of the entire health program; then he teaches you how to apply this knowledge and how to write your own special program. Then instead of making you write the computer program yourself, he surprises you and gives you a gift. He transfers a copy of a first-rate, time-tested program to you. He then allows you to link your own personal computer to the mainframe where all the knowledge of this health program resides. In this latter system, the energy connection between master and student is more important than postures. Using this kind of program saves enormous energy, which can then be directed towards self-healing.

This type of Qigong is very special because the master can use any object to pass healing Qi and messages to his or her patient. For instance, they can give a gift that carries this kind of message. The patient can then wear the gift, like a ring or necklace, and receive more healing benefits. The master can also use art, like painting, drawing or calligraphy. In this case, the master will give the patient a special piece of art that they can take home. Sometimes, a highly skilled master can use music for healing. This music is not like "New Age" meditation music, because when the master creates it, healing Qi is basically "channeled" through him or her for a very specific healing purpose, or even for a specific person and their condition.

Sadly, it is very difficult to find this kind of Qigong master today. From my experience, it's also difficult to find patients with an open mind who can accept this type of energy treatment. If however, the patient can open her mind, this is really the highest level of treatment she can receive. This is because she is being treated directly through healing Qi which reaches deeply into her body and mind. If she's treated with herbs, or acupuncture or acupressure, a transfer vehicle is involved. When that happens, there is an automatic step down or reduction in the percentage of the Qi or energy transmitted. Also, this type of treatment requires that the practitioner and patient form a deep energy bond.

Why are these kinds of Qigong masters hard to find? First these masters must have been taught by a skilled master. Their master must have trained them to discover this special gift. Second, even if they are lucky enough to meet a high-level Qigong master, if they haven't been born with the right energy structure or foundation to receive this gift, then the gift will never go beyond these masters. This concept becomes more clear when you think about how parents wish their child could inherit their own gift. Most parents would like to pass along their special talents to their children. But, even if a parent is a brilliant musician, they cannot make their child into one. The child has to have both the innate talent and the ability to receive the parent's gift. This gift is beyond technique and beyond words. In its simplest terms, it is an energy transfer.

The *Wu Ming* Meridian Therapy in our program falls into the second category of Qigong. It is derived from a very ancient system. Each of the movements has been selected for their ability to help stimulate Qi and help it flow in the meridians that run through your breast area. They are also designed to help you reawaken your natural healing ability. When you practice *Wu Ming* Meridian Therapy, you can get more benefit from working with the companion video to this book (See page 339 for more information.) It has been carefully designed from an energy standpoint. When you practice with it, you receive a strong Qi message that passes from me (in my role as Qigong master) to you through various energy waves that are set up to come from my physical demonstration of the movements, the visual picture, eye contact, voice wave frequency, and energy music that I created for this purpose. The more you practice, the more you will gain.

Chinese Psychology

Traditional Chinese medicine understands that balanced emotions are essential to well-being. Different excessive emotions, however, can cause the function of their corresponding organs to fall out of balance. If an illness is diagnosed as being caused by emotions, TCM believes that the best way to treat its root cause is to counter it with emotions. This seems logical enough, but has almost disappeared in practice. Here's how this works.

As we've seen, the five major organs—liver, heart, spleen, lung and kidney—are paired with their respective emotions—anger, joy, worry, sadness or grief, and fear or fright. And, as we've seen, each organ has two different relationships with the other organs: generation and control. The dynamic of control is the useful one in Chinese psychology. Here's a simple example: the liver controls the spleen. Because the liver's emotion is anger, its emotion naturally has control over the spleen's emotion, which is worry. Worry can be used to control fear. Fear can control happiness. Happiness can control sadness. Sadness can control anger. By studying the chart below, you'll get a better understanding of how TCM relates organs and emotions.

ORGANS	EMOTIONS	CONTROLS	ORGANS	EMOTIONS
Liver	Anger	→	Spleen	Worry
Heart	Joy	→	Lung	Grief
Spleen	Worry	→	Kidney	Fear
Lung	Grief	→	Liver	Anger
Kidney	Fear	→	Heart	Joy

Here are some famous ancient classical treatment examples I've selected to help give you a better idea of how this principle works.

❧Fear Fixes Excess Happiness

The ancient doctor known as the "King of Psychology" is Dr. Zhang Zi He (1156 to 1228 A.D.). One day, a patient came to him in desperation because he suffered from a condition of excess happiness. He could not stop smiling; his sleep was now disrupted, and he laughed constantly. He begged the doctor to treat him. Because of Dr. Zhang's reputation, the patient hoped he could be cured. On taking the case, the doctor checked his patient's pulse and suddenly had a sharp intake of breath. This sharp sound immediately alarmed the patient and made him think that his condition was quite serious. Dr. Zhang then told the patient that he had to leave to search for a very special herb. He left the patient and did not return for several days. During this time, the patient became increasingly worried. Finally, he became so convinced that he was so sick that he was going to die that he started to cry because he thought his condition was hopeless. He told his family that he would not be with them for very long. "My condition cannot be cured. I am certain that I'm going to die," he told them. When the doctor learned that his patient had reached this stage, he returned. He then reassured the patient that his condition was not as serious as he had thought. He gave him a simple herbal combination and sent him on his way. The problem was cured quickly. Dr. Zhang had used the technique of deliberately creating fear to relieve the condition of excess happiness. In other words, he had used the kidney's emotion to control the excess of the heart's.

✿Happiness Fixes Sadness

One lady-in-waiting in the Emperor's court had just heard that her father had been killed by thieves. She became so sad and cried so deeply that no one could console her. After her tears stopped, she began to feel a chest pain. Every day this pain grew worse. A few months later, it looked like a small ball had gotten stuck in her chest. Many doctors tried to treat her. No one could relieve her pain. Her family turned to Dr. Zhang and pleaded for his help. He came and immediately started to leap into the air, singing wildly, praying, and dancing around like a medicine man. Everyone was startled. This was totally unexpected and unusual behavior for the famous and dignified doctor. Because his movements were so silly and out of place, the lady-in-waiting could not help herself when she saw such amazing things. At first, she started to smile; then, she began to laugh uncontrollably. A few days later, the Qi stagnation that had created the lump under her chest wall was completely relieved. Here, the doctor used joy to overcome grief.

✿Anger Relieves Anxiety or Worry

A woman had to be separated from her merchant husband for several years because he had to travel far away on business. After some time, she began to worry about him constantly. She lost her appetite; she began to stay inside her home and never come out. She lost weight. Her family became very alarmed at her deteriorating condition. They asked many doctors to take her case. Each doctor tried his best to treat her with a wide range of special herbal formulas. None could bring back her appetite and she continued to lose weight and become dangerously ill. One day, Dr. Zhang passed through her town and her family begged him to help. When he found out the original cause of the woman's problem, he suddenly told the woman, "Why are you so upset over this man? I just heard he has found a very rich woman and plans to marry her." Once the woman heard this, she became so angry that she broke several dishes and stormed out of her house. A few hours later, she returned and still angry shouted: "I'm so stupid. How could I waste my love and energy on such a bad man." Then her appetite came back and she started to eat again. She began to recover her health. On his return through her village, Dr.

Zhang apologized to her and said: "I'm so sorry. I made such a bad mistake. The man I thought was your husband has the same last name as your husband and even comes from the same region. I hope you will forgive me." Dr. Zhang had used the technique of creating anger to resolve her anxiety.

❧Emotional Problems Cause Physical Ones

Here's how this concept appears in modern times. I've noticed that many of my women patients complain of chronic postnasal drip, which seems to be accompanied by a small lump in their throat. They usually blame their condition on sinus problems. The lump, however, is a very interesting one. They cannot swallow this lump, nor can they spit it out. They frequently clear their throat, or cough every few minutes. Some have even gone as far as having an operation on their nose. According to classical Chinese medicine, this is a well-known physical condition with an emotional cause. The ancient doctors even had a name for it; they called it *mei he qi*. Literally, these women have a lump of Qi stuck in their throats; the lump comes from chronic anger or sadness—a condition that the woman has not yet processed. This condition is so well known, that there is even a famous ancient formula to treat it. To fix the root cause of this problem, it is vital to rebalance liver function. No amount of treatment for sinus problems will ever solve this condition.

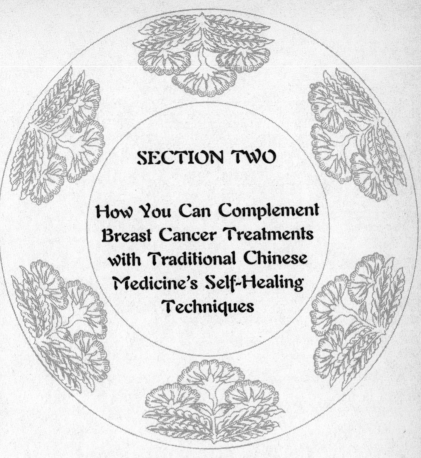

SECTION TWO

How You Can Complement Breast Cancer Treatments with Traditional Chinese Medicine's Self-Healing Techniques

The colors of the world blind human eyes;

The tones of the world deafen human ears;

The tastes of the world make human mouths water;

The pursuit of pleasures makes the human mind crazy;

The pursuit of the unattainable makes human conduct unnatural.

The wise man puts his ear to his heart and ignores his mind.

TAO TE CHING *(circa 500–200 B.C.)*

Υou now have a grounding in the basic knowledge of the principles, theories and techniques of traditional Chinese medicine. You now also have the information that allows you to make a connection between physical discomfort or external signs and an internal function disorder of one of your organs. Let me show you how to use TCM to help you complement breast cancer treatments.

Before you read further, please stop for a minute. I recommend you check yourself and see if your body has something to tell you. You'll find the early warning signs in Chapter 8 very important. You might want to reread this information at this point. If your tongue has ridges or edges around the side, if your tongue has a blue or purple mark on the sides, if your tongue has a thick white coating, if your nails are brittle and the half-moons have all but disappeared, according to TCM, you are already exhibiting the classical signs of a Qi deficiency and blood stagnation. If you are about to undergo breast cancer treatment, you should understand that you will need extra healing support because of the weakened energy condition in which you are starting treatment. You can also look ahead to the next section where there are healing foods and herbs, as well as healing recipes, that you can begin to apply immediately to build up your energy or Qi reserves.

CHAPTER 10

How You Can Trace the Root Cause of Your Breast Disease

THERE are many different kinds of breast disease. Fibrocystic breast disease is one common problem. It is so common, in fact, that Western medical reports say that more than half of all women have some form of this condition. The earliest reference to fibrocystic breast disease in classical Chinese medical literature appears about 300 A.D. during the Han Dynasty. The earliest reference in Western medicine was made by a Dr. Cooper in 1892. From the TCM perspective, this condition, like all breast diseases, is related to a liver function disorder. Because of its connection to the liver's function, it will naturally also be linked to the menstrual cycle. In the world of TCM, fibrocystic breast disease has its root cause in liver Qi stagnation. This stagnation is most often the result of emotional situations that cause chronic anger and stress (anger being the internal factor and stress the external factor that have the ability to disrupt smooth liver function). Often, this is the kind of breast disease that will take a quantum leap and develop cancer. Although Western medicine may suspect this is true, it does not have a comprehensive medical framework within which it can view the body, mind, and spirit as one holistic system that can correlate physical and emotional effects on a particular organ and its energy pathway to other critical body parts.

From centuries of successful experience, TCM understands that treating this condition early can help save the breast and prevent this condition from deteriorating. TCM doctors use acupuncture as well as the prescription of certain internal and external herbal formulas that have been specifically developed for fibrocystic breast disease.

There are many documented Chinese studies of successful treatment of breast disease. One interesting study done in 1982 by Dr. Cheng Jie Gou at the Shan Xi College of Traditional Chinese Medicine used acupuncture to treat five hundred women with a fibrocystic breast condition. The total effective treatment rate was 95.7 percent. These women received acupuncture treatment once a day with ten treatments equaling one course. Three to four courses were required. The effects of this method proved better than those in the control group treated with traditional Chinese herbs and Western drugs.

In another study, this same doctor used acupuncture alone to treat six hundred patients. Here the total effective treatment rate was 94 percent. TCM herbs alone have also proven highly effective in treating breast disease. One such study, published in 1981 in *The Journal of Traditional Chinese Medicine* (Issue 1; pg. 44), one of the most prestigious medical journals in China, describes a study of two hundred women treated for breast tumors with a special TCM herbal combination. In 177 women, the tumors completely disappeared. A different study, published in the same journal a year later by Dr. Gou, described the use of TCM herbs to treat 136 women for breast tumors. Eighty-nine were completely healed; thirty-one had a major improvement; six had some improvement; ten reported no benefit. The total effective treatment rate was 92.6 percent. In 1982, Dr. Wei Jun He published a report in the *Shan Xi Zhoun Yi Journal of Traditional Chinese Medicine* in which he described treatment of thirty-eight women with breast masses with an external patch of TCM herbs. Thirty-six women were completely healed after treatment.

As we've seen in Chapter 6, there are six major meridians that run through the breast area. Either a single meridian or a combination of meridians with Qi stagnation can cause a breast tumor or cancer. Generally speaking, most tumors or breast cancer develop in three distinct locations in the breast area. These areas are related to three major meridians—stomach, liver and kidney. There's a simple way for you to trace the meridian and organ related to your own condition. To understand this concept, let's use the clock as a reference point. Also refer to the diagram below.

The first sector is a straight line that runs from twelve o'clock to six o'clock, right through the nipple in the breast area. Any tumors or cancer growths that develop on this line are directly related to the stomach and its meridian, which govern

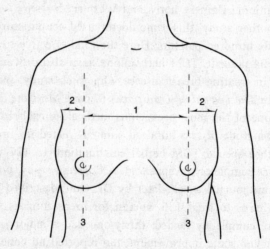

1. Related to kidney and liver
2. Related to liver and stomach
3. Related to stomach

this area (3). Any tumors that appear in the area between the two nipples are in the second sector. This inside area of the breast is related to the kidney and liver (1). Both organs influence this area's health; however, the kidney predominates. The other major sector that women should be concerned with is the outer area of both breasts (2). This is related to the liver and stomach; however, the stomach predominates. You can now use this knowledge to trace the origins of your breast disease to the major organ or organs that are its root cause.

As we've seen, from the TCM perspective, the definition of a healthy body is one where the organs function in harmony and Qi flows freely through the meridians. In this dynamic state, your body, mind and spirit are operating as one and tumors and cancer cannot develop. If this state becomes unbalanced from one or more of the many internal and external factors we've already identified, then tumors and cancer have an opportunity to incubate. Cancer's energy usually has a long time in which to find a place where it can safely hide in your body, root itself and begin to grow. During this time certain advance signs can appear to warn you of progressive imbalances.

I've listed many of them in Chapter 8 so you'll be able to recognize them and know how to interpret them, as well as treat them naturally with the TCM techniques and tools we've talked about. Again, the most powerful of these tools is *Wu Ming* Meridian Therapy. The reason I'm going over this information here is that, even though you may have been through surgery, chemotherapy or radiation (or any combination of these), you must understand that the root cause has gone untreated. This knowledge about the location of your breast tumor or cancer will allow you to trace it back to its root cause and the meridian and/or organ that is out of balance. You can then work at healing your specific root cause.

PRECONDITIONS THAT YOU MIGHT HAVE EXPERIENCED

❧ If your tumor or cancer is in any of these areas, think back before it appeared and try to recall some of the physical symptoms that TCM states are early warning signs. For example, if your problem is on the midline of the breast, your stomach was affected long before a physical mass appeared. Did you have frequent migraine headaches across your forehead? A bad taste in your mouth? Bad breath? Stomach distention or pain? Heartburn after you ate? Burping? Loose stool? Constipation? TMJ? Swollen gums? Did you lose your appetite? Were you depressed? TCM identifies these conditions as being related directly or indirectly to an imbalance in your stomach function. Remember that an imbalance means that the organ cannot perform its natural job or function. It does not necessarily mean the physical organ itself is diseased or has a problem. That is why your scientific tests may have been normal at that time.

❧ If your problem has developed in the second sector, it is related to the stomach and liver. Now, think back over time. Did you continually have cold hands and feet? Did you have PMS? Did you have irregular menstrual periods? Did you relate your anger to breast tenderness during your periods? Headaches on the side of your head? Frequent pain in the lower stomach? Frequent nightmares? Dreams of someone chasing you to kill you? Vaginal yeast infections? Mood swings? Did you become angry easily? TCM identifies these conditions as being related directly or indirectly to an imbalance in the relationship between the liver and stomach.

❧ If your tumor or cancer has appeared in the third sector, its root cause is a kidney function disorder. You most likely experienced a sequence of events relating to an imbalance in this organ. Did you feel cold inside all the time? Were you afraid of the cold? Did you have chronic lower back pain? Did you have urinary frequency or bladder infections? Did you lose hair? Did you have frequent vaginal discharge? Infertility? Did you feel frightened or panicked all the time? Lose sexual desire? Did you have chronic pain in your knee or your heel? Did your ears ring?

If you still have any of the conditions listed above, I recommend that you be very careful and take extra good care of yourself. The root cause of your tumor or breast cancer has not yet been healed. You should treat the source of the problem immediately. Take a look at Chapter 17 and identify the foods there that are good for the affected organ; practice *Wu Ming* Meridian Therapy at least once a day; review the herbs that relate to your affected organ. Find an acupuncturist or herbalist who will work with you to help you treat the root cause. Most of all, please look at your daily life. This is the most important advice I can possibly give you. Are you still doing the same things you did before you became ill? It is not necessarily a badge of achievement that you are able to resume your old life, though many will congratulate you on doing so. If you've been through breast cancer treatment, you've already had the strength to save your life once, I ask you not to go back to the same lifestyle that helped create a way for breast cancer to develop. Here is the crucial area where you can take responsibility for your own health and healing.

CHAPTER 11

Beginning the Journey: How to Handle Test Results; How to Find the Right Doctors for You; Ancient Self-Healing Techniques That Can Help You Successfully Prepare for and Complete Breast Cancer Treatments

THE information in this book can be used by everyone. If you do not have breast cancer, many of the self-healing techniques I've talked about can help keep your organs working in harmony and Qi flowing freely through your meridians. If you work toward achieving this state, TCM principles and theory state that you cannot get cancer. Adopt these self-healing techniques and you will have established a breast cancer prevention regimen that can protect your breast health. This is a proactive approach that is beyond breast self-examination. Remember that as important as breast self-examination is, it is early detection, not prevention. The actions in this book are preventive in nature; they were not invented a few months ago. They are based on time-tested, theory-based medicine that has helped literally millions of women for millennia.

If you've already been diagnosed with breast cancer, you

can benefit greatly from learning how to apply TCM knowledge to increase your physical and emotional strength. The result is you are able to prepare successfully for and complete your breast cancer treatments. If you understand from the previous chapter the root cause of your breast cancer and what you can do to correct it, you can keep your body healthy and help prevent a recurrence after treatments are completed. Let's look at what most women with breast cancer go through and TCM techniques you can apply to your own unique situation if you must meet these challenges.

HOW TO USE TCM TO MANAGE BREAST EXAMS

TCM, along with many other native healing systems, believes that the mind has far more power than the body. In my opinion, even though breast exams are important, especially for early detection, checking for breast cancer monthly and annually puts tremendous stress on a woman. This simple test forces her to think that she might be at risk for this terrible disease. I believe strongly that there is a way women can shift how they experience these checkups and turn them into positive, self-healing activities.

Monthly breast self-examination can be approached as an energy healing experience. Instead of worrying about where the cancer might be located, I recommend telling yourself instead, that wherever you touch, you are sending in healing energy to protect that location so that you will never have breast cancer. These powerful monthly mental messages can then work their way into your body, mind, and spirit. Early detection has helped many women save their lives. These tests and waiting for test results, however, can cause a tremendous amount of mental, physical, and emotional stress. As we have seen, unbalanced emotions can create or add to physical problems.

The challenge for women is to prepare themselves well to undergo annual mammograms and receive their results. My patients often ask me about these tests and whether or not they should take them. My response is that "If you are worried about getting breast cancer, then you should go ahead and have a mammogram. This will help eliminate negative thoughts." I also remind them "It's not what happens to you, but how you take it."

I then explain that before they take these tests, they should think about what the worst case for them might be. I ask them to take a moment to ask themselves these questions. If you already have a small tumor, what are you going do? Do you or don't you want surgery? If this tumor proves to be cancerous, what are you going to do? Are you going to have a mastectomy? Are you going to go to chemotherapy or radiation, or both? Do you have a doctor you know who cares about your breast instead of your cancer. Do you have a doctor who cares about your whole immune system and not just the cancer procedures? If you're asked to make decisions quickly, should you make them? Will you be able to keep your emotions under control and not panic? Can you allow yourself some time to reflect on what you are really willing to do? Naturally, you may not have the answers to all these questions, but at least you have given your mind a way to practice dealing with them, in the event something happens. Doing this exercise can help prepare the mind and cushion the very real shock of getting bad news about a mammogram.

If you believe you should undergo annual mammograms, then use the entire year to prepare your mind and body by working at prevention daily. Instead of worrying about these mammograms, you can look at the tests as confirmation that your own prevention program is working. Using this positive approach to handling annual breast exams is very important. I find that a lot of women become angry when they talk about mammograms because they feel they are looking for bad news. Many women also tell me how frustrated and frightened they are just to think about taking these tests. If you don't approach mammograms with a positive mental attitude, then the tests themselves can exert a certain kind of power over you and your emotions. Otherwise, these tests are almost like self-hypnosis where you think all year long, "I'd better go in for a checkup to see if I have cancer." Even though heart disease is the number one killer of women, most don't walk around telling themselves, "I better go in for a checkup to see if I'm going to die from heart disease." When you repeat this kind of message constantly, you are actually giving yourself very powerful, yet subtle programming.

Think about it this way, do you go to your local police station each year to check your fingerprints and to see if they belong to a criminal? No, you know who you are, and you know that you have not committed a crime. There are people in the world who do commit crime, but you know, with 100 percent certainty, you are not one of them. I am not advising against mammograms or monthly breast self-examination, because we know they do help women. What I want women to realize is that there is a positive, proactive way to use these tools so that they can get maximum healing benefit from them. I want them to recognize that they can choose not to create negative mental programming that can affect the body, mind and spirit.

I would like everyone who reads this to understand just how powerful their mind is. Recently, some amazing work on the body and how it responds to placebos has been done. And there are a number of studies that have already shown that those who actually deny they have cancer, live longer than those who accept the reality of their cancer. Why? Quite simply, the power of your mind is much greater than the power of your physical body. When your mind is in complete denial, it helps your body create an energy defense system to fight with the cancer. There are many interesting scientific studies that confirm the power of the mind-body relationship.

HOW TO HANDLE TEST RESULTS

According to TCM theory, the root cause of breast cancer lies primarily in Qi stagnation, which is always related to emotional factors. Being diagnosed with breast cancer is in itself a highly emotional, stressful, and frightening moment. It is important to know that, at this time especially, any excess emotional Qi you expend can actually aggravate the root cause of your condition. As difficult as it may be, it is vital to keep your emotions stable and not let this negative information destroy your hope of healing completely. You will need all the positive emotional, mental, physical, and spiritual energy you can create over the course of your treatment to conquer cancer's energy pattern. It is this accumulated Qi or healing power that you will use to help heal yourself. From this very moment, you must remind yourself daily how important it is to save your Qi for the big healing work ahead.

After being diagnosed, many women run themselves ragged going from specialist to specialist to obtain more information and more opinions. This can be a confusing effort and a big drain on Qi. Although you may feel the need to take immediate action, there is almost always enough time to help yourself regroup your emotional, mental, spiritual, and physical energies. Based on experience with my breast cancer patients, I know that stopping to take this simple step of integration can make a tremendous difference in the outcome of your treatments. Many women feel this research effort is important; if you go through this step, just remember to take time out to listen to your intuition.

We've described how to prepare yourself for getting the results of breast cancer tests. When my patients have been diagnosed with breast cancer, I recommend they also take a little time to calm down so they can think about what they want— not what other people want. I would say to you, if you were my patient, think about what you want to do, what you're willing to do, and what you are able to do. Try to understand your current mental and physical condition. Given whatever condition your body, mind, and spirit are in, is it reasonable to expect yourself to handle the treatments being proposed? Remember, there will be more difficult steps in this journey. Try to work with doctors who have a desire to treat you as a whole person. Try to use the least invasive procedures possible. For example, TCM believes that lymph nodes are very important to overall health. If you don't have to excise them, then leave them intact. Deciding on treatment is a critical juncture; some women already become overwhelmed and give up their healing power at this stage. They may end up going through the treatment steps, but they've already abandoned hope. Because their mental state has changed, they cannot unite their body, mind and spirit to fight with cancer effectively.

Remember, too, that no matter what kind of doctor or what kind of treatment you choose, you are the one who must eventually fight with cancer's energy pattern. Developing a strong will is critical. Facing breast cancer is like fighting a war with an unknown enemy. You must take the time to analyze its strengths and weaknesses so that you can create a plan that allows you to control or kill this enemy. Starting from strength can make all the other steps much more productive.

HOW TO FIND THE RIGHT DOCTORS FOR YOU

TCM believes that the most successful treatment occurs when the energies of the patient and the doctor are in harmony. It sees this healing work as a partnership. In TCM theory, the patient is not merely a passenger and the doctor the driver; rather, they are partners who have joined together to fight illness or disease. For this reason, finding the right medical and surgical partners is one of the most critical steps in fighting breast cancer.

The right partner is not necessarily the most famous doctor, or the busiest doctor, or the one who treated your friend. You should seek out a doctor with a passion for caring about you personally and for your problem individually. You should tune into your intuition and see if you have a good feeling about this doctor. Because TCM believes that part of the root cause of breast cancer comes from Qi stagnation caused by excess emotions, it is important that you choose a doctor who is empathetic and will take your emotions and emotional concerns seriously, as well as help you address your emotional needs. Also, choose doctors who will honor your beliefs and respect your intuition. Remember the final fight is yours. The doctors can only assist you. The *Nei Jing* tells us, "Your life belongs to God; Your health belongs to you."

Ask your doctors how many of the procedures they recommend they have performed. Ask them their overall philosophy of health and healing. What is their opinion of the effect of the mind on the body? Do these doctors believe in complementary medicine? Will they work with you if you choose to use it? Ask them how much time, in general, they can spend with you when you are scheduled for a visit. Find out if they can refer you to a support group. I have had the privilege of working with SHARE, a well-respected New York City self-help organization for women with breast or ovarian cancer. We have been using the *Wu Ming* movements outlined in this book for a five-week course for breast and ovarian health. There are a number of other self-help organizations throughout the United States that you can contact. Also the worldwide web provides many sites that offer some helpful information. The Susan G. Koman Foundation has a very good one at www.komen.org. Our center also has one for TCM at www.breastcancer.com.

Using the guidelines for choosing a TCM practitioner we discussed in Chapter 9, I recommend that you also find a local herbalist and acupuncturist to complement your breast cancer treatments. Using Eastern and Western medicine together to combat breast cancer has proven very effective in China today. In fact, classical Chinese herbal formulas are one of the few treatments that can actually increase T cell counts between chemotherapy or radiation treatments. And, these herbal formulas also offer one of the few effective treatments for relieving the side effects of chemotherapy and radiation. Remember to consult the healing recipes in Chapter 17. A number of them are also good for alleviating side effects.

CHAPTER 12

Surgery: How to Prepare Yourself With TCM Techniques; How to Use TCM to Undergo Surgery; How to Help Yourself Complete Breast Cancer Treatments; How to Help Yourself Recover

*B*EFORE surgery, TCM has several things you can do that can help make your surgical experience more successful and recovery more rapid. I always review these principles with my patients so that they understand how they can maximize their healing opportunities. Remember TCM believes that we are woven into the greater Universe and that we can connect with its energies to help us heal. To follow are a number of things you can do for yourself.

Time

TCM believes that the precise time at which you are born is the time your body's Qi is most strongly connected to Universal Qi. This influence remains with you your whole life. Consequently, if possible, you should choose to have surgery at your birth time so you can receive maximum support from Universal energy. If this is not possible, then see if you can have your surgery scheduled during the morning hours. At this time, earth Qi is rising and gaining strength. By matching with nature's Qi, you can help strengthen your own. The days before and during the new moon or the full moon also are better energy choices than other days. It's interesting to note that ancient doctors were very mindful about how time of day and time of season affected healing opportunities. Their treatment times were scheduled around what was best for the patient. It is hard to imagine finding this kind of attention in our Western culture.

Herbs

When I first began working with patients with breast cancer, I would give them a special herbal combination that they could cook themselves at home. Later, I created a number of special herbal combinations in capsule form to support people through various phases of breast cancer treatment. These classical herbal combinations are all based on ancient formulas; I adapted them for Western patients. This is a very important aspect of these herbal formulas, because we talked earlier about how Chinese medicine treats an individual patient according to "who you are," "where you are," "when you are," and "how you are." In the case of my patients, I need to take into account the "where" of Western society and its constant stresses. I developed one herbal formula to be taken before and after any surgery; another is good for relieving the side effects of chemotherapy or radiation. The third has been adapted for my Western patients to help them increase Qi and strengthen the body's overall function. (For more information on our TCM herbal formulas and teas, contact our Traditional Chinese Medicine World Foundation. You'll find the address in the back of this book.)

Any surgery can deplete your body's Qi and blood, so it is important to get as much extra healing help as possible before and after surgery. In China today, many doctors who practice

Western medicine for breast and other types of cancers, combine it with TCM herbs because they are so effective in helping strengthen the immune system and in increasing T cell counts. This benefits the patients by allowing them to remain strong enough to complete a course of cancer treatments successfully. For example, at Beijing Hospital, 134 patients were treated for breast cancer with chemotherapy and radiation. They were also given a TCM herbal formula to help strengthen their immune systems. Five years after this combined treatment, 88.8 percent of these women were alive. In another study at the same hospital of patients with several different kinds of cancers, more than 85 percent of patients given a combination of chemotherapy and Chinese herbs were able to complete a full course of treatment; in the control group without herbs, only 19.4 percent were able to complete treatment.

Foods

TCM uses foods before surgery to help strengthen the body's blood. At this time, eat as much spinach and red beets as possible. Seafood like shrimp, lobster, clams, oysters, and mussels are also a good addition to presurgery meals because they have the ability to strengthen your kidney Qi. Any kind of bone marrow or bone marrow soup can also help increase blood volume and help make you stronger overall. Eat as many of these foods as often as possible in the weeks before your surgery.

Rest and Meditation

It is impossible to overstate how important it is to rest before surgery. Resting recharges your energy and helps your body and mind come together so you can undergo surgery successfully.

Most women before breast surgery are already exhausted mentally, emotionally and physically. According to TCM, this state causes your Qi, or healing energy, to flow erratically all over your body. If you undergo surgery at this time, you will have more difficulty recovering. Instead, rest and meditation help the body collect its Qi and center it. This can protect you from losing excess Qi during the operation. I strongly recommend you take care of your mind, as well as your body, before any surgical procedure. Find the time to meditate quietly as often as you can. During your meditation, call on your deepest healing ability and give yourself the most positive healing messages possible. Think of your immune system and its strength; think of yourself as a powerful energy being who can heal herself. Above all, think about how you will totally cure yourself after surgery. Feel this surge of positive energy run through your whole body and do your best to keep these positive thoughts with you at all times.

HOW TO HANDLE BREAST CANCER SURGERY THE TCM WAY

On the day of your surgery, try to keep your emotions as stable as possible. I know this is easy to say, but very difficult to do. However, knowing the importance that stable emotions play in helping control breast cancer, you should make every effort to remain peaceful. The more calm and peaceful you are, the more Qi you will be able to save to protect and heal yourself later. Make sure you eliminate everything and everyone who does not support this critical step.

Before surgery, take slow, deep breaths and concentrate your attention on your navel. Focusing on this special Qi point can help your own Qi remain powerfully concentrated in your core. This step can help you conserve more energy to recover faster. As the anesthesia begins to work, you are unconsciously giving yourself a strong, positive healing message.

HOW TO HELP YOURSELF RECOVER FROM BREAST CANCER SURGERY

After surgery, there are many more challenging steps to come that will create demands on your mental, emotional, and physical energies. To successfully weather the breast cancer treatments ahead, I ask my patients if their doctors will allow them to take a short rest before undergoing chemotherapy or radiation immediately. I advise them to use this time to recover and rebalance their Qi for the next part of this journey.

Once again, it is essential to rest . . . rest . . . and rest some more. Many of my Western patients are programmed to keep "running on empty." In fact, they don't even know they're "on empty." Our society is one of action and activity that rarely sees rest as productive. Nothing could be farther from the truth—especially when it comes to healing your body! As I do with all my patients, I ask you to give yourself permission to rest. Here again is another vital area where you can take responsibility for your own health and healing. Resting is one of the easiest and best ways to preserve and build up your healing Qi. Eat the same foods before treatments that are recommended above before surgery. Work with a knowledgeable herbalist. These steps can help boost your body's healing Qi to a higher level so you are ready for the next stage.

CHAPTER 13

How to Manage Your Health During Chemotherapy or Radiation

*B*EFORE you undergo chemotherapy, radiation, or other breast cancer treatments, consult with the doctors you trust. I advise my patients to choose a treatment based on their breast cancer's needs rather than on automatic medical protocols. You must really understand each step of a proposed treatment, what it does, what you will get, and what demands it will place on your body's energy. You must also understand the condition a given course of treatment will leave you in if, for some reason, you're unable to complete it. Again, take time to calm yourself and become peaceful and clear so that you can make the wisest choice—the one that suits your own unique mind, body, spirit, and emotions. Use your intuition; try to choose the treatment with the least side effects. Remember that you will need your healing Qi for the challenging steps after treatment.

As everyone knows, there are many side effects from various breast cancer treatments: hair loss, nausea, joint pain, insomnia, loss of appetite, and constipation to name a few. All of these conditions are symptoms signaling the deeper acute Qi dysfunction or crisis from which your organs are suffering. It is important to emphasize that TCM has treated these kinds of

Qi dysfunctions effectively for centuries; it offers a number of ways to help you rebalance your body's overall function, accumulate healing Qi, and help reduce side effects from these treatments.

To complete these treatments successfully, your body will use up tremendous amounts of Qi. Some Qi will also be consumed by the activities of your daily life; additional Qi will be used up to fight with the side effects of chemotherapy or radiation. You can see how critical it is to rest so that you can build up your reservoir of healing Qi. If possible, I recommend that at the beginning of these treatments you reduce your work schedule and cut down on the number of things you do. Even if you feel you still have energy, I recommend you save this energy for your own self-healing. Frankly, I ask you to be very selfish in how you spend your Qi or vital energy. Become conscious of the choices you make every day. For instance, does it make sense to use up invaluable Qi by spending three or four hours shopping? Or going back to an eight-or nine-hour workday? In general, avoid any strenuous activities or exercise. Have sex in moderation.

Some TCM herbal formulas can help your body relieve the side effects of chemotherapy and radiation and help you go through these treatments more successfully. I use a combination of two unique herbal supplements, which are based on famous ancient recipes used safely and continuously for hundreds of years. Many doctors and hospitals in China today use variations of these famous formulas to help hundreds of thousands relieve the side effects of breast cancer treatments. They also help patients accumulate enough strength to successfully complete treatment.

MENTAL PREPARATION

Because breast cancer treatments can compromise your immune system and cause multiple side effects, you may experience a great deal of physical discomfort as well as overall Qi deficiency. These problems can ultimately affect your mental state. Please remember that no matter how difficult it is for your physical body to undergo breast cancer treatments, you must never give up hope. TCM believes that your body always has a chance to heal itself. Your mental belief can either strengthen your body's energy function or cause it to collapse. The interlinked system of mind and body is never more important than at this juncture. It is essential to maintain the strongest mental outlook you possibly can. Keep your energy focused on the positive aspect of getting well; do not burn up your healing Qi with negative thoughts.

As you undergo chemotherapy or radiation, you can tap into the power of Universal energy by imagining that you are under water and that the moon is shining above your head. Here you are using the power of your own healing Qi to counteract the intense heat of treatment. Imagine you are receiving the cool and healing yin energies of the moon. After chemotherapy or radiation, you should imagine you are receiving the sun's warming yang energies and that they are destroying cancer cells. Imagine the sun is beaming healing Qi deeply into your body. This effort is beyond visualization. Remember we talked earlier about the ancient principles of yin and yang—two complementary, yet opposing, natural energies. Here we are applying the yin/yang principle to help your body come into balance and derive more support and strength from the Universe.

Here is a description from one of my patients about her experience combining Western breast cancer treatment with TCM practices:

"I was fortunate at the time of my breast cancer diagnosis several years ago, because I was both a patient and a Qigong student of Dr. Lu. Looking back, I find it difficult to imagine that devastating period without the support of his acupuncture and herbal treatments, as well as his guidance.

As a Western woman I chose to follow a course of standard Western cancer treatments—but I did it with a very important difference. I followed a course of Eastern treatments at the same time. Eastern medicine strengthened my Western treatments because it strengthened me. And isn't this what is missing most from Western medicine? As patients undergoing cancer treatments, we hand over all our personal power to a team of medical experts, machines, and drugs. The result is that we begin to feel a little less like ourselves each day. Paradoxically, the same doctors pat us on the back and tell us how important a positive attitude is for our survival, yet nowhere in our experience with Western medicine is there anything that empowers us to feel that way.

But my experience was different. Through traditional Chinese medicine, I learned to believe in myself as a self-healer who could use the power of her mind and body working together for her own recovery. This was most dramatically demonstrated to me by my experience with TCM and radiation treatments.

The week prior to beginning radiation I was having acupuncture treatment and Dr. Lu asked me what I was going to think about during my radiation sessions. I answered that I would probably envision a relaxing, soothing beach scene with me being nourished by the sun. He said, 'Please don't do that. You will burn.' When I asked him what I should think about, he said, 'The opposite. Focus on the Moon and feel yourself protected by her cooling tides.'

When I got to the hospital the next week, they were indeed concerned about my highly reactive skin, which made me even more nervous. But each day for eight weeks,

I remembered Dr. Lu's advice and took the Moon into the radiation room with me. Day after day, I imagined her and her cooling tides in there protecting me. I knew I was safe and would not burn. And I didn't. Not at all. Not even during the week of 'boost' treatment which was directly over my nipple. The doctors and technicians were very surprised. My skin did not burn or change texture, and due to Dr. Lu's other treatments, my energy remained high throughout. All atypical results, which I can only attribute to what I was doing differently through Eastern medicine."

FOOD

According to TCM theory, the side effects of chemotherapy and radiation are the result of the lung, stomach, and kidney functions becoming seriously deficient. It is important at this time to include foods in your diet that help support the health of these organs. While undergoing cancer treatments, I recommend you include as much fresh fruit and lightly cooked vegetables as possible in your diet. I do not recommend eating raw vegetables. The reason is that during this time your digestive system is already being weakened by the cancer treatments. In TCM's view, eating raw vegetables consumes extra Qi for digestion and will overwork your digestive system. Though you might lose a little nutrition by cooking vegetables, you will conserve more Qi for healing. You will also help strengthen your stomach's function. (Remember we said the stomach "hates" to receive cold things!)

The healing energies of "live" or fresh fruits and vegetables can help all the major organs recover more quickly. A few foods deliver more healing benefits than others do. For instance, eat as much of the following as possible: pears, almonds, kiwis, dandelion greens, carrots, and sugar cane juice. Add clams, mussels and oysters as often as possible. These foods are particularly effective for reducing internal heat caused by radiation or chemotherapy. American ginseng and gingko biloba are the only two herbs I recommend taking individually (see Chapter 17 for more information on classical Chinese herbs).

ENERGY PRACTICE

The *Wu Ming* Meridian Therapy in this book can help restore the free flow of Qi or vital energy throughout your body—particularly in the meridians or energy pathways and organs that relate to breast cancer. These ancient energy movements can be performed by anyone at any stage of breast cancer or breast cancer treatment. They can help your body, mind, spirit and emotions become one so you have more power to recover rapidly. See Chapter 16 for a description of these movements. Practice them as often as possible. You can also practice gentle exercises like yoga and Taiji.

Walking is usually very good for everyone who has undergone breast cancer surgery. Walking slowly and thoughtfully can help make your Qi flow smoothly through your body and lets you tune up with nature. Again, you can get more energy by tapping into the Universe by connecting with nature. Enjoy being in nature, whether in the forest, in the park, at the seashore, or in the mountains. Wherever you are, try to merge or flow with nature's healing energies. I do not recommend fast walking (or jogging, or aerobics) for any of my breast cancer patients because it uses up too much Qi—this is Qi that should be conserved for healing. If you've had your lymph nodes removed, try to raise your arm very slowly each day as often as you can. Even though this may be painful at first, you will be helping to reestablish the flow of blood and Qi through this area. The first two movements of *Wu Ming* Meridian Therapy are especially good for helping you recover a full range of motion in your arm.

Here are some comments from another of my breast cancer patients:

"I started working with traditional Chinese medicine about one month after beginning chemotherapy for breast cancer. My hair had fallen out and I was wondering if I would have enough energy to continue working while I was on chemotherapy. I began to have treatments once a week of acupuncture and Chinese herbs. After about two months, while in the middle of my six-month chemo treatment, I was surprised, and so were my doctors, to see my hair begin to grow back. By the time I had finished the chemotherapy, my hair was long enough for me to stop using wigs and scarves. My energy levels remained high enough so that I was able to maintain a normal schedule of activities, both career and social. Since completing chemotherapy, I have continued with acupuncture and Chinese herbs. I also began a program of *Wu Ming* Meridian Therapy. Today, I actually feel healthier, with higher energy levels, than I did before being diagnosed with breast cancer."

CHAPTER 14

Beginning the Real Healing Work: Why and How to Create a Lifestyle Plan with TCM to Address the Root Cause of Your Breast Cancer

PERHAPS the most difficult time for breast cancer patients is after treatment. You may have finished seeing your doctor regularly; you may be finished with your support group, and you may now have started a long-term drug regimen like tamoxifen. Often, at this time, women feel lost; they feel like they are on their own. I hope you will view this period as your opportunity to begin the next and most critical stage of your self-healing journey.

You can be happy you've successfully completed surgery and/or treatments for breast cancer. Remember though, you now must address the root cause of this problem to truly heal. As we've said throughout this book, according to TCM theory, breast cancer is caused by Qi stagnation in your meridians, or energy pathways, as well as the dysfunction of one or more of your major organs. Unless these deeply rooted conditions are addressed and rebalanced, your body is susceptible to cancer's energy pattern. This pattern has found a comfortable match with your own, and is intelligent enough to hide in your body until conditions are favorable again for growth. Unless you totally change your lifestyle, your emotional reactions, your thought patterns—unless you change your energy pattern from the inside out—you are leaving yourself vulnerable to this disease and others. This is one reason why breast cancer patients can find themselves battling cancer later in their life.

From the TCM standpoint, it is important to understand that after chemotherapy or radiation, your body is still not fully recovered. Your body, mind and spirit have undergone a great deal of stress and you are still in a somewhat weakened state. Even if you feel good mentally, your internal Qi still needs attention. At this time especially, you should do everything in your power to take good care of yourself. Slowing down can actually help you recover as quickly as possible. Whatever you do, I urge you not to go back to your "old life." Do not go back to your old energy patterns: lifestyle, emotions, habits, and the like. Consider yourself newly born! To reach this stage, you have already experienced using your healing ability. Yet, there is more work ahead. You can help yourself truly and deeply heal, if you are willing to make the necessary changes.

To prevent a recurrence of breast or other cancers, you will need to do two specific things: keep your body and Qi foundation strong; look at your lifestyle and make positive changes. When you make these changes, your own energy patterns will also change. This will make it harder for disease to remain or enter. Even after you've completed chemotherapy or radiation, it is vital to continue complementary treatments. Remember at this point, the damage that chemotherapy and radiation have done to your body will take some time from which to recover. Your complementary treatments can help you build Qi for self-healing.

Another thought I'd like to pass on to you: TCM theory states that it is possible to live a long, healthy life with illness or disease, as long as they are kept under control. It does not believe in absolute "kill." Remember the example of the famous treatments for parasites we discussed. This treatment (and many others), used for thousands of years, is based on this theory. The herbal treatment basically puts the parasite to sleep, thereby stopping its breeding and eating patterns; the host is left untouched. TCM applies the same theory to breast cancer. Strengthening and altering your internal energy pattern can control cancer's own pattern. The result is that you are unlikely to die from breast cancer itself.

After breast cancer treatment, one of the most common drugs prescribed is tamoxifen, an antiestrogenic agent. Often, women are on this drug for at least two years and up to five years. At this time, studies show tamoxifen to be helpful in the treatment of breast cancer. However, tamoxifen, either in combination with chemotherapy or alone, can produce a number of side effects, some of which are similar to the natural energy transition of menopause: hot flashes, night sweats, vaginal discharge, and dryness, gastrointestinal symptoms, depression, thromboembolic effects, uterine malignancies, and ophthalmologic symptoms.

While tamoxifen symptoms are similar to menopausal symptoms, their root cause is different. Menopause is a natural, usually gradual, transition; however, many women experience uncomfortable symptoms because their overall Qi (especially kidney Qi) is stagnating and deficient. With tamoxifen, the body is suddenly thrown into an unnatural, chemically induced, menopausal condition. These symptoms are especially difficult for the premenopausal woman and can cause serious discomfort.

Unfortunately, if you're taking tamoxifen, you do not have the option of using hormone replacement therapy (HRT) to relieve its side effects or symptoms. TCM has successfully helped treat menopausal symptoms for many centuries. In fact, more than a thousand years ago, a famous formula for hot flashes was already in common use and continues to be used to this day. I believe TCM has much to offer women who are being treated with tamoxifen.

From my own experience, TCM can offer substantial relief to women undergoing menopausal symptoms, whether from natural or drug causes. I know that women taking tamoxifen can benefit greatly from applying TCM theories and techniques and practicing *Wu Ming* Meridian Therapy. It is not a matter of choosing between Eastern and Western treatments, because TCM can be used successfully alongside tamoxifen therapy. If you are taking tamoxifen, you can help yourself on this part of your healing journey. First, incorporate *Wu Ming* Meridian Therapy movements into your daily routine. These ancient energy movements can make a major difference in the way you feel. Be sure and communicate with your doctor, or other health workers, let them know all the things you are doing to help yourself heal.

I recommend that you take the time to answer the questions in the self-healing checklists in Chapter 15. They are very important and will help guide you and give you an understanding of the TCM point of view about specific healing lifestyle changes you can make in eating habits, work environment, emotions, sleep routine, among other things. Each answer offers knowledge about how to conserve your Qi, or vital energy, to keep it strong and flowing freely.

After chemotherapy or radiation, your biggest challenge is to prevent a recurrence of breast cancer or any other catastrophic illness. The medical treatments you've undergone have only treated your cancer. They have not touched the root cause. Now it is your responsibility to treat the root cause of your breast cancer. Don't think that because you have successfully completed these medical treatments that you can resume your old ways. If you do, you are definitely at risk for breast cancer's return. It is your old lifestyle that produced this breast cancer in the first place. You now literally have a new lease on life. I believe that everyone has something that they were born to do; your successful survival of breast cancer means that you have been given more time to complete your life's mission. Try to do something you love; try to let go of everything that causes you pain, stress, anger or sorrow. After reading this book, you should have a very good idea of how these emotions affect the way your physical organs function. Do your best to alter your former life patterns so that you eat, sleep, work and play for healing. Do your best to really connect with the endless loving energy of the Universe.

If there is one final thought as you undergo the challenges of breast cancer treatment that I would like to send deep into your consciousness, it is that you have been born with the ability to heal yourself. My wish is that traditional Chinese medicine helps you discover this extraordinary gift.

TCM TIP FOR SELF-HEALING

- ❧ Keep your emotions peaceful and stable.

- ❧ Practice *Wu Ming* Meridian Therapy.

- ❧ Eat for healing.

- ❧ Take healing herbs.

- ❧ Monitor your self-healing progress with our TCM form.

SECTION THREE

Prevention is the Real Cure: How You Can Help Yourself Heal, or Prevent Breast Cancer or Its Recurrence with Traditional Chinese Medicine

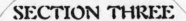

The best doctor concentrates on prevention instead of fixing disease.
The wise doctor concentrates on bringing the whole body into harmony instead of fixing its imbalances.
If you're already sick and then begin medication,
If your health is already out of control and then you start to address it,
You are like a thirsty man digging a well, or a soldier making his weapon in the midst of battle.
You are too late.

NEI JING (475–221 B.C.)

When I talk with women about breast cancer, I usually get many of the same questions before I launch into an indepth explanation of traditional Chinese medicine. From group to group, these questions reflect a belief on the part of these women that breast cancer has an external cause. Naturally, this prompts them to search for an external cure. Some will ask: What about the environmental factors? What about the chemicals I encounter? What about the sun damage I had when I was a teenager? What about the fact my mother and aunt had breast cancer? What kind of foods will cure my breast cancer? What kind of herbs can eliminate my breast cancer? Can Cat's Claw help? Will shark cartilage prevent cancer? Can't soybeans cure or prevent cancer? And more. All these questions are rooted in the same thought—"Somewhere, somehow, there is something out there that can help cure me or prevent breast cancer." All these questions are not necessarily wrong, but they have missed the main point. They have not focused on the fact that their own body has developed the breast (or any other) cancer. And that they have the ability to treat small physical conditions before cancer progresses to an acute stage where surgery, chemotherapy or radiation appear inevitable.

TCM specializes in prevention. In this paradigm, prevention means creating a totally healthy body and totally healthy lifestyle. This is lifelong work that gives the individual an excellent chance of living a healthy life of good quality. Contrast this with our modern society where we tolerate many different seemingly minor health conditions and still call ourselves healthy. For instance, look how many people experience fatigue at 3:00 in the afternoon. Their eyes cannot open and their mental function is just about gone. Normally, this is the body's sign that you need to rest and recharge yourself. But we don't or can't listen to this simple basic message. So, what do we do? We use cups of coffee or cigarettes to stimulate us. Or, let's go back to the car analogy. If you drive really long distances, you know that it's a smart thing that after a number of hours you should stop and give both the car and yourself a rest. You know that pushing it could be dangerous. Now suppose you push your car harder and the light for overheating comes on, what do you do? Usually at this time, most people would stop and let their engine cool down or rest. Then they would add water. You know that if you continue to drive with an overheated engine, you will almost certainly experience dangerous and expensive problems. Like the car, we also have many warning signals that advise us of more serious internal problems ahead, but often we ignore them or override them with things like coffee, cigarettes, aspirin, or sheer will power.

In Chapter 15, I have created a series of key checklists that will help you understand certain physical conditions that are your body's warning signs, which according to TCM might lead to more serious health problems in the future. I've also included information on essential things you can do for yourself to prevent your energy from being completely depleted or situations that deplete your Qi. With this knowledge, you can hold the power of real prevention in your own hands.

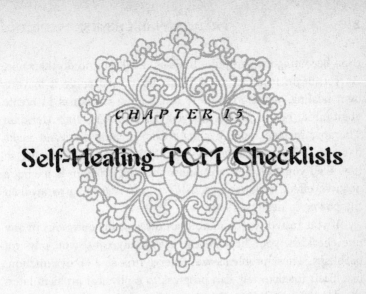

CHAPTER 15

Self-Healing TCM Checklists

*A*s we've discussed, TCM understands that the root cause of breast cancer is stagnation of Qi in one or more of the six meridians running through your breast area and an imbalance in one or more of your body's organs. TCM states that when Qi runs smoothly through the meridians and the organs work in harmony, good health can be maintained. There is no way for disease or illness to enter this well-operating whole system.

The following self-healing checklists are an essential part of a TCM prevention program because they allow you to discover where Qi stagnation may develop and which of your organ(s) may be out of balance. They also provide a blueprint for positive steps you can take to help prevent conditions that can lead to the root cause of breast cancer. Many seemingly common or "inconsequential" women's conditions are, in reality, internal messages signaling an energy dysfunction which, as we have seen, can progress to breast cancer. It is very important to pay attention to these signals and habits that can unbalance your Qi or vital energy. Whenever I speak to women, whether they're patients, students, or new audiences, I tell them to take these signs seriously so that they can prevent minor health problems from becoming catastrophic illnesses. I ask you to do the same. As you begin to understand TCM theory and apply it to your own healing, work with these self-healing checklists to create your initial health profile. As you perform *Wu Ming* Meridian Therapy, include more healing foods in your diet, and make daily lifestyle changes, you will gradually notice a difference in how well you feel. You will know that the program is having a positive effect. Congratulations! You are beginning to awaken the power to heal yourself!

If you answer yes to more than three of the questions in any one checklist, your lifestyle can eventually cause you physical problems. These problems will emerge first as a Qi dysfunction, but if left uncorrected, can progress to a physical problem later. (Look back and review the Breast Cancer Progression chart on page 18.) According to TCM theory, there are many ways you can conserve Qi—the healing energy you will need to help prevent a recurrence of breast cancer, help you through breast cancer treatments, or prevent breast cancer's energy from taking hold in the first place. Making positive changes in your lifestyle can yield tremendous healing benefits for longevity. I have set up six separate checklists. Look over the answers and, where possible, try to make the necessary changes they suggest. You can coordinate this knowledge with the *Wu Ming* Meridian Therapy, the energy massage instructions, and healing foods and herbs in Chapter 17. With these tools, you can design your own program and take charge of your healing process.

I. SELF-HEALING CHECKLIST FOR EATING HABITS

Taking Care of Your Digestive System

7. Do you eat barbecued or fried foods often?

2. Do you always drink ice-cold drinks or ice water, particularly during your menstrual cycle?

3. Do you eat raw vegetables or eat at salad bars frequently?

4. Do you get a headache after you have a meal?

5. Do you experience stomach distention whenever you eat?

6. Do you have a stomachache after you eat, particularly after eating cold or dairy foods?

7. Do you always burp or pass gas after you eat?

8. After you eat, do you always have loose stool when you go to the bathroom?

9. Do you drink too much alcohol? More than two glasses a day?

10. Do you have food allergies?

ANSWER SECTION ON EATING HABITS

A function disorder in your stomach will cause the stomach's Qi to stagnate in your stomach meridians. From an energy standpoint, it is essential to keep your stomach functioning well. Fifty percent of breast cancer cases develop in the upper outer quadrant of the left breast, a location that TCM understands as being related to stomach meridians. Therefore, keeping this organ functioning properly is essential to keeping Qi flowing freely in this critical breast area.

1. Barbecued or fried foods can cause a stomach function disorder by creating an excess of heat in this organ. This condition of internal heat can be compared with the kind of heat a compost heap gives off. It is a kind of intense, inner smoldering that then prevents the stomach from performing its normal job—one aspect of which is to work in harmony with the liver. According to TCM, the stomach and the liver must have a healthy partnership to digest food well. The stomach meridians

run down the front of the torso (in line with the nipples) through each breast.

2. The stomach's very nature is warmth-loving. Warmth then is the natural law on which this organ operates. It "loves" to receive warm things like soup, tea, etc. If you constantly eat or drink cold foods or beverages, you can unbalance the stomach's natural function and cause it to perform sluggishly. If you eat and drink cold things during your menstrual cycle, your liver and uterus might draw this cold energy to them. This, in turn, can cause cramps, an irregular cycle, or other types of female problems. Switch to warm liquids and foods with a warm essence, which can be found in Chapter 17.

3. Many Westerners believe that eating raw vegetables provides better nutrition. TCM believes that raw vegetables have a cold essence that is not naturally good or supportive of the stomach's function. Even though you might get a little more nutrition from raw food, you will expend more Qi to digest it. If you cook a vegetable slightly, you may loose a little bit of nutrition, but you will save a lot of Qi that could better be diverted to healing and protecting your stomach function. I believe this information is especially important to women undergoing breast cancer treatment because they need every bit of healing Qi they can conserve.

4. The stomach meridians run up through the forehead area. Generally speaking, headaches in the front of the forehead that occur after a meal indicate a stomach Qi deficiency because the stomach is drawing on too much energy to digest its food.

5. Stomach distention means that you are suffering from a stomach Qi deficiency. It also indicates that your liver is not working in harmony with your stomach. As we've noted, digesting food well depends on a good partnership between these two organs. Stomach distention means they are not supporting each other's function. Too much stress usually causes this kind of discomfort. Learn to be peaceful before you start a meal.

6. As indicated in answer 2, the stomach's nature is warmth-loving. If you get a stomachache after you eat cold foods, your stomach's Qi has become unbalanced and is now too cold. This is a signal that you should change your eating habits immediately and switch to giving the stomach warm foods or foods with warm essence (like ginger, cinnamon, scallion, and fennel). These foods can help relieve this kind of stomachache. Look at the list of foods in Chapter 17 for other choices.

7. Burping or passing gas after you eat indicates that the stomach's Qi is deficient. Your organ does not have enough Qi or vital energy to work at its assigned task of digestion. If this happens after you eat raw vegetables, cheese, or other dairy products, or when you're under stress, it is a sign that your stomach and liver's partnership is shaky. Again, this is a signal that they cannot function in harmony with each other.

8. Loose stool after eating means that the stomach and spleen both have a Qi deficiency. This crucial organ pair can not operate efficiently. Your digestive system is weak. Avoid cold foods; substitute warm foods.

9. Excess alcohol will cause the liver's Qi to stagnate. If the liver's Qi stagnates long enough, it will affect the stomach's Qi and cause a disruption in communications between these two organs. Again, here is a lifestyle habit that has the potential to seriously unbalance the harmony between these two vital organs. When this happens, your digestive system suffers. It then becomes difficult to derive enough Qi and nutrition from any foods you eat to support your body. Most people do not understand that in order for foods, vitamins, nutritional supplements, or even drugs to work on the body, they must first be processed by a properly functioning system that comprises the stomach and the liver. There is virtually no way to extract the nutrients you need from whatever you put into it if the processing plant itself is not working.

10. Food allergies are an indication that your stomach Qi is low or deficient. They also mean that your stomach cannot work in harmony with its liver, spleen, and gallbladder. Many people, in an attempt to address their allergies, gradually cut out one food after another in their diet in the hopes of relief. Sometimes, I see patients who are basically down to eating rice cakes and water because they have become so sensitive. They are so focused on believing that their problem is caused externally by the foods themselves, that they are literally shocked when I tell them it is their stomach that is the problem. Changing your diet alone does not get to the root cause of this problem. Avoiding cold foods, raw foods and ice-cold liquids may help significantly. Adding warm foods and foods with a warm essence like ginger and cinnamon can also help. I urge you to study the foods in Chapter 17 and start adding the appropriate ones to your diet. This can make a big difference in your life if you suffer from food allergies. So can practicing *Wu Ming* Meridian Therapy.

II. SELF-HEALING CHECKLIST ON SLEEP HABITS

1. Do you have difficulty going to sleep each night?

2. Do you wake up at the same time each night? What time?

3. Do the same dreams recur frequently?

4. Do you have nightmares?

5. Do you experience night sweats?

6. Do you go to bed after midnight?

7. Do you eat a big meal and then go to sleep?

8. Do you have to take a sleeping pill or other drug to sleep soundly?

9. Do you get up to urinate frequently during the night?

ANSWER SECTION ON SLEEP HABITS

Sleep is the state in which both your physical body and its energy system take a rest and regenerate themselves. During this time, your body's Qi is recharged—much like a battery. If you sleep well, your body is ready to go with a new charge. If you do not sleep well and wake often, you have less Qi or vital energy to get through your day. TCM examines your dreaming to diagnose the quality of your sleep. For example, if your body is in deep harmony, your sleep will be quite deep, and you should not consciously remember your dreams. You still dream, but these dreams are not accessible to your conscious mind. TCM also uses dream interpretation to understand the energy condition of your various organs. (Chapter 8 describes how this information applies to understanding breast cancer.)

1. If you have difficulty falling asleep continually, generally speaking, your spleen and heart Qi or energies are deficient. This means these two partners are not functioning in harmony. Remember in our discussion of balance and harmony, we said that the state of harmony reflects one dynamic system that has a smooth, automatic, unconscious exchange of energy. In this instance, your spleen and heart are out of sync. Your mind cannot calm down long enough for you to fall asleep. If you toss and turn during sleep, the cause is the same. Slow breathing or meditation before you go to bed can help.

2. TCM theory states that Universal energy changes every two hours and your body's meridian and organ energies respond to and match these changes. For example, energy changes start with the lung, which is "on duty" or in charge of the body from 3:00 to 5:00 A.M. If your lung's Qi has a problem, then you might find yourself waking up in this time period. Or, you might wake up with a physical problem like a cough during these hours. Here are the other times of Universal energy changes and their related organs:

Lung	3:00 A.M.–5:00 A.M.
Large intestine	5:00 A.M.–7:00 A.M.
Spleen	7:00 A.M.–9:00 A.M.
Stomach	9:00 A.M.–11:00 A.M.
Heart	11:00 A.M.–1:00 P.M.
Small intestine	1:00 P.M.–3:00 P.M.
Bladder	3:00 P.M.–5:00 P.M.
Kidney	5:00 P.M.–7:00 P.M.
Pericardium	7:00 P.M.–9:00 P.M.
Triple warmer	9:00 P.M.–11:00 P.M.
Gallbladder	11:00 P.M.–1:00 A.M.
Liver	1:00 A.M.–3:00 A.M.

3. Dream diagnosis or interpretation is one tool TCM uses to understand a patient's physical condition. Qi problems in the internal organs show up in different kinds of dreams. For instance, if your heart Qi is deficient, you might feel yourself falling out of the sky or off a tall building. If you have a kidney Qi deficiency, you might have dreams that are connected to drowning or being under water, or being in a boat that is capsizing. Or, you might find yourself being fearful and hiding from something in your dreams. If you refer to the Five Element Theory chart on page 84, you can see where this insight comes from. Water is the element of the kidney and fear is its ruling emotion. You can gain more insight into your dreams by studying the Five Element Theory chart. If you always see yourself arguing or fighting or things are destroyed in your dreams, then you might have a parasite, or these could be signals that your internal problem might be worsening.

4. Generally speaking, nightmares indicate a liver Qi deficiency—nightmares that contain images of people chasing you, wanting to kill you, or harm you usually indicate a problem with unbalanced liver Qi. If you have these kinds of nightmares,

your liver is in need of attention. If these dreams occur frequently, your body is sending you stronger signals that the liver needs your help. According to TCM, the liver is the most important organ for women's health. I recommend that you pay serious attention to these kinds of internal warnings. Remember if Qi stagnates in the liver or this organ becomes completely out of balance, you are looking head on at the root cause of breast cancer.

5. Sweating at night indicates that your body's yin Qi is deficient. This means that at nighttime, your body's Qi cannot control the normal opening and closing of the pores in your skin. One of the key principles of TCM is that the body has two types of energy—yin and yang—that must work in harmony. Daytime Qi is considered yang; nighttime Qi is yin. If you have more physical discomfort in the daytime, your body's yang energy is deficient or is not sufficient enough to handle normal daytime tasks. The reverse is true if your problems occur at night.

Also, if you experience night sweats during chemotherapy, radiation, or tamoxifen therapy, this means that these treatments are having a serious effect on your yin Qi. This is a sign that you should add things like clam juice or oyster juice to your diet. Adding ginseng in any form can also help you. Special classical Chinese herbal formulas can stop this problem and help ease you through these treatments. These combinations are in widespread use today in China in conjunction with Western-type cancer treatments.

6. It is important to understand this from an energy perspective. Your body enters its yin Qi phase after midnight—the body's energy moves deep into the internal organs to rejuvenate them. To remain in harmony, your body should follow nature's way. If you stay up past midnight, you are working against nature's cycle and will spend more than twice the Qi needed

for every hour you're awake just to stay awake. To save your Qi or vital energy and prevent disease or illness, it's important to follow nature's cycle. This is especially critical if you're undergoing cancer treatments since they are already depleting your body of precious Qi, which you need for self-healing. Get to sleep, if possible, before midnight. Try to get a good eight hours of restful sleep to help yourself heal.

7. Many Western people eat a big dinner and then go to sleep. This often causes sleep problems. TCM understands that insomnia is often related to different types of stomach Qi problems. When you eat a big meal, the stomach's energy will overfunction or work too hard. By overworking, it can fall out of harmony with the liver and heart. (Refer to the Five Element Theory chart to see the kinds of relationships among these organs.) That's why some people feel heartburn after a big meal; however, the root cause is often a dysfunction of the stomach's Qi. Healthy eating means that you should only eat to about 70 to 75 percent capacity of your stomach. Eating too much before bedtime means that your stomach must use extra Qi to function all night long just to digest what you've eaten, when it should be conserving this Qi for self-healing and resting. Here again is another simple, yet effective, way to build up your Qi or vital energy and not waste it.

8. TCM understands that sleeping well means your body is functioning in harmony. If you always rely on sleeping pills or drugs, your body cannot function in harmony. Also, these substances might be hiding a deeper internal problem that needs to be fixed. I recommend that my patients try to find other natural ways to help them sleep better.

9. Urinary frequency during the night indicates your kidney Qi is deficient. This means that your kidney cannot send your bladder enough Qi to hold your urine throughout the night. If this condition occurs during or after cancer treatments, it means your body's overall Qi has dropped significantly. Classical Chinese herbal formulas have been used successfully to help this condition without interfering with the cancer treatments.

III. SELF-HEALING CHECKLIST ON WORK HABITS

1. Do you work in or around high-power electric areas or where there is radiation such as a microwave?
2. Do you work with chemicals?
3. Do you like your job?
4. Do you work under chronic stress?
5. Do you work straight through your day without taking a lunch break?
6. Do you work and eat at the same time?
7. Do you get along with the people you work with?
8. Is your work area comfortable and healthy?

ANSWER SECTION ON WORK HABITS

If you have breast problems or breast cancer, you should understand that you are different. It is your old lifestyle that has contributed to this problem in the first place. Often my Western patients are eager to "get back to their life." I tell them this is a concept they should reconsider very carefully. I urge them to change their habits and their emotional responses to the stress in their lives if they truly want to heal and address the root cause of their breast cancer. Likewise, if you want to prevent breast cancer, then you need to understand how you can change your daily work habits so they do not deplete your Qi or vital energy. Understanding the effect of your work environment on your health is a very important aspect of self-healing.

1. Electrical fields can interfere with or change your body's own electrical field. New scientific work with bioelectromagnetics at Stanford University in California shows that even very subtle frequencies far below what was considered safe can create cellular changes. Electrical fields can cause a dysfunction in the flow of Qi through your meridians. They also have the ability to cause a serious Qi deficiency. The stronger the field, the worse the effect. If you work around a radiation area, your immune system could become weakened by this kind of energy force. If you are continually exposed to these kinds of energies, you are at risk for compromising your own self-healing ability.

2. Certain kinds of chemicals can either directly or indirectly cause cancer. Even if you don't directly touch the chemical, simply smelling it can interrupt the smooth and healthy functioning of your lung. According to TCM theory, the sense organ associated with the lung is the nose. Additionally, the lung controls the health of the skin. If your lung function is interrupted, then your skin can be affected.

3. Because you spend the largest part of your day at your job, you invest a lot of emotional, physical, mental, and spiritual energy there. If you don't like your job but you must keep it, then your mind and spirit are in conflict and under constant pressure. This condition can cause internal Qi stagnation in any organ or meridian—which is related to the root cause of breast cancer. If you always find yourself in this situation, physical problems will eventually show up somewhere in your body. For instance, during the menstrual cycle, you may experience PMS, headaches, sleep problems, breast tenderness, and so on. You may not relate these symptoms to chronic emotional discomfort or distress, but according to TCM theories, this is the root cause of the physical discomfort.

4. Stress takes a deadly toll on the liver, which is the most important organ for women's health. If your liver function is out of balance, then you might experience physical discomfort in the form of symptoms such as menstrual disorders, PMS, stomach distention or bloating, nail problems, and itchy and/or red eyes. If the liver continues to be stressed over time, this condition can lead to function disorders of other critical organs, such as the stomach, kidney, heart, and lung. It is vital to find a healthy way to deal with the stress in your life. It is important not to absorb the negative energy of stress into your own energy system, but find productive ways to let it go. TCM has a time-honored and very successful way to alleviate anger: smash eggs! In fact, buy a dozen eggs (a pretty inexpensive way to let out stress) and smash them all. Believe it or not, this simple act can help you physically and emotionally relieve a lot of anger and stress. Some of my patients come back to me and say "Why didn't you tell me to get two dozen eggs!" They love this therapy. No eggs? Try smashing raw potatoes with your feet (shoes on!). Or, in a safe place, break glass bottles. The results are remarkable.

Acupuncture, yoga, and meditation, and certain Chinese formulas can help relieve stress, as well. Our *Wu Ming* Meridian Therapy movements are especially effective at helping you reduce chronic stress in your life. Here again having the discipline to practice the healing movements is another opportunity to take control of your own health.

5. Because of the multiple lives women lead today, they often work long, stress-filled hours, sometimes forgetting to stop for lunch. This causes the body to expend or burn up extra Qi for daily activity. When this happens, your body is forced to draw on your irreplaceable kidney Qi to keep going. This is not a good situation because we've seen how instead it should be running on the Qi of your rechargeable stomach energy to get through the day. Not eating healthy foods at regular intervals will cause a stomach function condition that could eventually

lead to digestive system problems later like food allergies, bloating after eating, and weight gain. Again, continuing this unhealthy habit can lead to more serious digestive problems when the stomach becomes unable to extract nutrition from the things you eat. A stomach organ problem could disrupt the healthy flow of Qi through the stomach meridians, which run through the breasts. An energy blockage in this area could create a mass or worse. Help yourself by taking the time you deserve to eat at regular intervals in a peaceful environment. Even if you take only twenty minutes, you can help yourself tremendously.

6. Working and eating at the same time is not a healthy habit. Each activity draws on its own separate energy source. If you work and eat at the same time, then your digestive system does not get sufficient Qi to do its job. You may not be able to gain maximum nutrition from the food you're eating while you're working. If you always do this, then you can literally upset or unbalance the normal functioning of your stomach. Then, you may experience stomachaches after eating. Because 50 percent of breast cancers appear in the area through which the stomach meridians run, it is critical to do everything you can to keep this organ and its meridians functioning well. This is true prevention.

7. While you don't have to love the people you work with, it's very important to have a harmonious work experience. Otherwise, your body will spend extra Qi to deal with emotional issues on a daily basis. This emotional discomfort can cause a function disorder of one or more organs. Go back to the Five Element Theory chart on page 84 and review which emotions can affect which organs. According to TCM theories, the root cause of breast cancer is closely related to holding unbalanced and/or negative emotions in the body. Held over time, this negative energy can stagnate and cause serious damage. It is not the experience of the emotion that is damaging—this is only being human. It is the chronic holding of the negative emotion that causes problems of stagnation. To remain well, it is important to find healthy ways to release excess emotions from your body and become good at "letting things go."

8. Again, because you spend so many of your waking hours in the workplace, it is very important to create harmony in your environment to the best of your ability. This way your body does not have to divert extra Qi just to maintain its normal function. Even a few small changes can help you conserve Qi. When a plant flowers, it is at the peak of its energy. Try to bring a fresh flower often into your workspace to experience nature's special Qi. This kind of "live" message can help your body recall its own healing energy. Place an evergreen plant near your computer. When your eyes become tired, change your field of vision to the plant. This can help you relieve eyestrain and help keep your vision healthy. Everyone can take a few short breaks during the workday. When you do, close your eyes and breathe slowly and deeply. Let everything go; do not focus on any problems or physical sensations or emotions. I tell my patients that even a few minutes done throughout the day can really help them recharge their energy base. Many short meditations can produce the same effect as a full twenty minutes of meditation. Getting into this habit can change your life and help you accumulate tremendous health benefits.

IV. SELF-HEALING CHECKLIST ON EMOTIONAL STABILITY

1. Are you depressed? Do you take medication for depression?
2. Do you suffer from angry moods continually?
3. Do you cry easily very often?
4. Do you suffer from anxiety or panic attacks?

5. Is it hard for you to make decisions?
6. Do you worry all the time?
7. Are you under a lot of stress for continued periods of time?
8. Do you suffer from frequent mood swings?
9. Do negative events from the past continue to bother you today?

ANSWER SECTION ON EMOTIONAL STABILITY

TCM believes emotional problems are directly related to the root cause of breast cancer. Different emotional problems will cause different organs to experience a function disorder. For example, TCM believes the liver is related to the emotion of anger—too much anger held for a long period of time can affect the liver's function and the way it performs the tasks it's programmed to do. Overthinking will cause stomach and spleen function problems, sometimes manifesting as a loss of appetite or excess water retention, respectively. Healthy lung function can be destroyed by chronic sadness. A continual state of fear will compromise kidney function. And too much joy or too much happiness will ultimately cause a heart function problem.

1. TCM understands depression as a disharmony between liver and spleen Qi. If you use drugs to help alleviate depression, you may have a temporary lifting of the condition but the underlying root cause is still there. Similar to pushing a ball under water, sooner or later the problem will pop up again unless this root cause is fixed. TCM understands that treatment of this problem means addressing both the unbalanced internal Qi condition and the emotional reaction to external factors that cause this illness. It is important to identify why and how this problem has come about. Though drugs for depression have helped many people through many difficult times, they can eventually cause liver and stomach function problems.

2. Anger will cause a liver function disorder. TCM understands that the liver is the most important organ for women's health. Because the liver is responsible for the smooth flow of Qi and blood throughout the body, a liver function disorder can also affect other organs and cause them to become out of balance. If this happens, you might experience problems such as nausea, cramps, headaches, and breast tenderness during your menstrual cycle. If the anger becomes chronic, then the liver's function will deteriorate and Qi can stagnate in its meridian. These are the root causes of breast masses or uterine tumors.

3. Crying is related to the lung function and sometimes the stomach and spleen functions. Crying all the time can weaken the Qi of all three organs. They will then not be strong enough to keep their ruling emotions stable nor will they be able to help keep your overall emotional energy stable. Excess sadness can weaken your immune system.

4. Anxiety and panic attacks are related to deficient kidney Qi. These conditions can also mean that your kidney and heart are not functioning in harmony. Because the kidney is the major energy source for the entire body, the best way to address these conditions is to treat the root cause by increasing kidney Qi with Chinese herbs.

5. TCM understands that the gallbladder rules the body's decision-making capability. If your gallbladder Qi is deficient, or the gallbladder itself has a function disorder, you might have a hard time making decisions. If your gallbladder has been removed, you might also find—especially as you get older—that making decisions becomes difficult.

Sometimes, gallbladder problems are also related to a liver function disorder. If you're under a lot of stress, or if your liver does not function smoothly with its companion organ, the gallbladder, or with the other organs, then gallbladder function will be impaired. Also, if you have digestive problems, such as difficulty eating protein or dairy products, the root problem lies with the gallbladder.

6. Constant worry can cause spleen and stomach function disorders. If that happens, your digestive system will be affected. Your body will not be able to extract enough nutrition from what you eat, you might experience lack of appetite, you might retain water, and your sleep may become disturbed. Conversely, if your spleen Qi becomes weak or deficient, you may begin to worry constantly.

7. Stress is the number one external emotional cause of liver function disorder; anger is the number one internal emotional cause. Unfortunately, many women today are affected by both of these conditions. If there is a liver function disorder, then you're very likely to have a digestive problem. The consequence of this is an internal Qi crisis. When this crisis occurs, your whole body's energy system can become deficient or weak. The body lacks enough power to support its everyday functions. It starts "running on empty." This, in turn, causes more stress as you become increasingly unable to handle basic daily activities. Chronic stress can actually be deadly. It can cause serious Qi stagnation in the meridians or the organs. Chronic stress causes most of the health problems many women experience today. TCM believes that, for women, as long as the liver function remains in harmony, then breast cancer can be prevented. That is why I warn my patients that they must look at their lives seriously and try to eliminate stress and anger wherever possible. This is real prevention. *Wu Ming* Meridian Therapy can help by bringing the body, mind, and spirit into harmony. Practice this ancient, self-healing system as often as possible.

8. If you suffer from frequent mood swings, particularly before your period, or at menopause, or after cancer treatments, two key organs are affected. Your liver Qi is stagnating (the concept of stagnation is like that of a compost heap, which generates a kind of smoldering, internal heat that blocks the free flow of Qi) and your kidney Qi is weak or deficient. Acupuncture and Chinese herbs are very successful treatments for these kinds of problems. Taiji, yoga, meditation and relating to nature's energy by walking can help you regain your emotional balance.

9. "Letting go" is one of the most important philosophies of TCM, which uses many different techniques to push disease and illness out of the body. These include: treating a cough to expel it from the body instead of suppressing it, or using herbs to put a parasite to sleep instead of trying to eject it with harsh chemicals. And, when it comes to cancer, one of the major TCM treatments involves strengthening the immune system so that it creates an energy field stronger than the cancer itself within which it can be contained. TCM prefers not to use up the body's finite Qi reserves to fight head on with the cancer, but rather to focus on helping the patient live a long life—in many cases alongside of the cancer itself. This approach is used successfully in China to treat cancer patients.

As a method of treatment, TCM tries to relieve or unblock Qi stagnation. If you always mull over the past, replay distressful scenes, reflect on past negative events and feelings, hold grudges, or never forgive, sooner or later this stuck energy, or Qi stagnation, can turn into a physical blockage, like a tumor or cancer. If you want to heal yourself, completely letting things go is the only way to change your body's energy pattern—no matter what problem, the technique is the same. Disease or cancer is a type of energy formation that has chosen your body as a place to stay for many years. It will not leave its comfortable host easily. If you have trouble letting past negative emotions go, imagine how much more difficult it will be to find the strength to let cancer's energy go.

V. SELF-HEALING CHECKLIST ON PLEASURE HABITS

1. Do you have to be in constant motion?
2. Do you overeat?
3. Do you smoke?
4. Do you drink too much alcohol? More than two glasses per day?
5. Do you have frequent sex, or frequently change sex partners?
6. Do you perform high-impact exercises more than three times a week?
7. Do you take drugs, either prescription or recreational drugs?
8. Do you take birth control pills?

ANSWER SECTION ON PLEASURE HABITS

1. If you're always in constant motion, you are using up a lot of excess Qi to support your physical and emotional activities. The body is much like a car. It needs a rest; at regular intervals it needs its engine turned off and it needs to cool down. Also, like a car battery, the body needs to recharge itself. According to TCM theory, everyone is born with a finite amount of Qi. If you constantly consume large quantities of Qi, it hastens the time when this finite amount is completely depleted; in other words, it's time to die. It may appear that you're accomplishing a lot of things when you're in constant motion, but in reality, you may not be doing the best job, or even the highest quality work. You may be in motion without reason. You may tend to become frustrated more easily, which might unbalance your liver; this in turn will set off a negative cycle that can lead to more serious health problems. When your Qi level falls too low or weakens, you are more vulnerable to becoming sick and you do not have an adequate reserve of Qi to

heal yourself. Learn to say "enough" and give yourself permission to slow down and make intelligent choices about how to use your time and energy. I realize this is particularly hard for women to do because of the many demands placed on them. I remind my patients that making healthy choices is the most important thing you can do for yourself and your loved ones.

2. If you continually overeat, you can cause a serious stomach function disorder. Your stomach will become distended; you might experience heartburn. Overeating will also cause your body to spend much more Qi to digest what you've eaten. According to TCM, stomach dysfunction can also cause insomnia. Often, sleep problems are caused by eating a big meal too late at night. If you have this kind of problem, don't take sleeping pills. Shift your eating habits and avoid eating or drinking too much before bedtime. Healthy eating means eating enough not to feel hungry later. This requires tuning into your body's signals so that you can recognize what a satisfied feeling means for your body. I recommend my patients eat to about 70 percent of the capacity of their stomach. Not eating too much will also help your mental function. It can help you think more clearly and eliminate a sluggish feeling.

3. Everyone knows that smoking is harmful to your health. Cigarette smoke will not only cause lung cancer by affecting this organ and its meridian, but it will also affect your large intestine and kidney meridians and the actual organs themselves. Remember that your lung and large intestine share a partnership and communicate through Qi. Smoking can cause large intestine and kidney function disorders. If these two organs are out of balance, you will gain weight after you've quit smoking because both of these organs, which have the job of ridding the body of excess water, have also been thrown out of balance. Remember that the tissue of the lung is the skin. Smoking will also compromise your skin quality.

4. Everyone knows that excessive drinking can cause liver problems. However, according to TCM, the liver has additional and very different functions than it does in Western medicine. For women, if the liver is out of balance, it will affect the stomach's function and cause menstrual cycle disorders and emotional problems. If liver problems continue, you might eventually experience Qi stagnation in the liver meridian. This meridian runs through the breast area. Other symptoms of liver Qi problems include breast tenderness before your periods, headaches on the sides of your head during your menstrual cycle, continual stomach bloating, bad breath, and a red nose (which is due to excess internal heat in the stomach).

5. In TCM's view, too much sex will cause liver and kidney Qi deficiencies. You might experience a lot of vaginal discharge. If it worsens and becomes yellow or burns and itches as well as takes on a bad odor, you might then experience ringing in the ears, hair loss, and lower back pain. If you really overdo sex, you can even experience eye problems. If you are undergoing chemotherapy or radiation, you definitely need to have sex in moderation—for instance, about once or twice a month. This will help you conserve your Qi for self-healing purposes. Changing sex partners frequently also uses up too much liver and kidney Qi and can cause additional problems. You also might contract a sexually transmitted disease if you do not protect yourself. Naturally, if you have other health problems, this can seriously compromise your efforts to get well. Here's another area where smart, responsible choices can help you heal.

6. Many women have been told that they are doing the right thing by exercising vigorously—that high-impact exercise will help protect their cardiovascular health. TCM regards exercise differently. First of all, the body is approximately 70 percent water. A water type of body needs water-type exercises to match its energy frequency. Also, TCM theory states that the liver governs the tendons. High-impact exercises often cause tendon problems that, in turn, can affect the liver and create a liver function disorder. That's why some women who overexercise do not menstruate. They have a liver dysfunction that impedes the free flow of Qi and blood in their body. I see a lot of chronic fatigue syndrome patients—almost all of them have a history of overexercising, especially with high-impact aerobics. I recommend soft exercises like dancing, yoga, Taiji and, of course, noncompetitive and gentle swimming, which matches well with our "watery" bodies. One of the best exercises of all is slow, gentle walking in nature, where you can tune up your body, mind, emotions, and spirit with nature's healing energy. I recommend being fully present in nature—don't wear earphones, don't carry weights, don't speed walk. If you want to test your cardiovascular condition and go beyond the physical level, pay particular attention to the last movement in our *Wu Ming* Meridian Therapy. The longer you hold this posture, the more benefit you will gain for both your heart and your lung.

7. If you're a frequent drug user, whether nonprescription or prescription, it's likely that your symptoms are being addressed instead of their root cause. Most drugs are constructed in such a way as to suppress a problem instead of healing the root cause. All drugs are toxic to some degree; they must all eventually be processed through your liver. For your own health, you need to identify the root cause of your problem instead of continually addressing its symptoms. Sooner or later, the health problem you believe you're treating can emerge in another part of your body. Just like holding a ball under the water, sooner or later, when your strength cannot hold the ball under water any longer, it will pop up. While you're under drug treatment, you can also look for complementary treatments that can help strengthen your Qi, so you might be able to reduce your drug dosage. This way, your immune system can become stronger and allow your own natural healing ability to take over.

8. Birth control pills affect the liver, the most important organ for women's health. TCM believes that unless the liver functions in harmony with your other organs, you cannot get pregnant. To help women who have difficulty getting pregnant, TCM treats the liver and coaxes it back into balance. Because birth control pills suppress your ability to become pregnant, they also suppress your liver's function. Women who have been on birth control pills for many years often experience difficulty getting pregnant because their liver function has become impaired.

VI. SELF-HEALING CHECKLIST FOR FREQUENT DISCOMFORTS

1. Do you suffer from PMS?
2. Do you suffer from hayfever?
3. Do you suffer physical symptoms when the weather or the seasons change?
4. Do you frequently have bad breath?
5. Do your ears ring?
6. Are your nails brittle or cracked?
7. Is your nose area red all the time?
8. Do your eyes tear frequently?
9. Do you have frequent headaches?
10. Do you suffer from adult acne?

ANSWER SECTION ON FREQUENT DISCOMFORTS

1. TCM understands PMS as a symptom of a liver function disorder. PMS is not in a woman's mind. PMS encompasses a wide range of associated problems, such as many different types of headaches including migraines, nausea, constipation, loose stool, anger, depression, mood swings, among others. The root cause of all of these seemingly unrelated conditions is the same—liver Qi stagnation. As long as the liver function disorder remains untreated, these problems will remain. I often see patients who regard PMS as simply something they must put up with, uncomfortable as it is. I really try to educate these women about this condition and what a serious warning sign it is. I urge you not to ignore any PMS symptoms.

2. Hayfever usually occurs in the spring and fall. According to TCM, if an organ's energy function cannot match a season's energy change, then you will become sick. Spring is the season of the liver, and the eye is the "window" of the liver. If you get hayfever in the spring, you might have the most trouble with itchy, watering eyes. Fall is the season of the lung, and the nose is its "window." Accordingly, if you get hayfever in the fall, you might experience the most trouble with a runny nose. No matter what season, if your organs are out of balance with the energy change, you will most likely experience some kind of health problem. Fixing the organ's function is the way to permanently address this problem; covering up the symptoms with medications is only a temporary measure.

3. If your body's Qi or energy is not in harmony when weather or seasonal changes occur, your body will produce different kinds of health problems. For example, if your body has too much dampness or maintains a lot of water, then when it's damp or the rainy season comes, you may experience arthritic pain. If you always catch a cold or the flu in the winter, the season that the kidney rules, your condition is related to a kidney Qi deficiency. If you experience headaches at the top of your head or excessive anger or mood swings when winter turns to spring, your liver function is out of balance. If you have heart problems or heart disease, you might experience a lot of discomfort in the summer whose ruling organ is the heart.

4. Bad breath is one indication that the body has liver Qi stagnation. This condition can, in turn, cause your stomach Qi

to overheat. Emotional problems or stress can bring this kind of bad breath on. Mouthwashes, toothpastes, and breath mints will not address its root cause. Look for healthy ways to relieve any emotional discomfort especially if it is chronic. For instance, TCM has one way to reduce stress. Buy a dozen eggs and smash them. Or, smash raw potatoes by stomping on them. Or, in a safe place, break glass bottles. Though these actions may seem a little unusual, they are time-tested TCM ways to help relieve anger. Fried, barbecued and/or spicy foods can generate excess heat in your stomach which, in turn, can also cause liver Qi stagnation. Try to avoid these foods whenever possible. Make sure you have regular bowel movements.

5. If you do not have a physical problem with your ears, ringing in the ears means you have a kidney Qi deficiency. You should regard this as a serious health sign because, according to TCM, the kidney is the body's Qi or energy foundation. There are certain foods you can add to your diet to help strengthen kidney Qi. Eat clams, lobsters, oysters, shrimp, black beans, walnuts, and other nuts as often as possible. When this condition persists, TCM treats it with herbs or acupuncture.

6. TCM believes that you can identify internal conditions by examining external signs. For instance, your nails are the mirrors of your liver. If your liver is healthy, your nails should be shiny, grow fast, and not break easily. If your nails are in poor condition and crack or break easily, you must treat the liver. Gelatin, shellfish, and clams can help your nails improve. Examine your nails periodically; if the half moons are not white and full, your liver Qi is weakening or becoming deficient. Take care of yourself; this is an early warning sign of internal imbalances.

7. In TCM theory, if the nose area is red, then the stomach is suffering from excess heat. This condition is also sometimes related to unbalanced liver function. Unless the condition is fixed from the inside out, most treatments are temporary. Acupuncture, herbs, and lifestyle changes can help alleviate this condition.

8. The eyes are the "window" of the liver. If your eyes tear frequently, or if you wake up with matter in your eyes, your liver Qi is stagnating. A liver Qi dysfunction has now progressed to a physical problem. It is important to treat the root cause of this condition before it progresses further and reaches more advanced stages. Refer to exercise #6 in Chapter 18 (pg. 317) on healing gates. Acupuncture, herbs, and lifestyle changes can also make a beneficial difference.

9. According to TCM theory, six different meridians with yang Qi or energy run through the head. Qi stagnation in one or a combination of these meridians can theoretically cause 720 different kinds of headaches ($6 \times 5 \times 4 \times 3 \times 2 \times 1 = 720$). To effectively treat a headache, it is essential to identify the organ that is out of balance. For instance, headaches on both sides of the head relate to the gallbladder; headaches at the front of the head relate to the stomach, and headaches at the top of the head are associated with the liver. Taking painkillers may alleviate headaches temporarily, but they can mask more serious problems that can emerge later. As you can see, headaches are merely symptoms telling you that there is a deeper problem, which resides in one or more of your five major organs. You can also see that headaches are specific to the individual. Your husband's headache may be different from yours, as yours may be different from your mother's. That is why pain relievers only work for some people some of the time.

10. If you suffer from adult acne, TCM theory states that your liver and kidney organs are out of balance. The messages that they need to exchange to keep your skin clear and unblemished are not being communicated properly. Unless you restore balance in this important relationship, it is unlikely that your acne will improve permanently with topical treatments. TCM believes that it is essential to treat adult acne from the inside out. Chronic anger and stress are two of the major causes of this condition.

CHAPTER 16

Wu Ming Meridian Therapy: Ancient Energy Movements You Can Perform Daily for Self-Healing

*T*HE most important part of our Nine-Point Guide to Self-Healing with TCM (in Chapter 4) is the *Wu Ming* Meridian Therapy. I have developed these exclusive, unique ancient energy movements with my master, Professor Xi-hua Xu of Yunnan, China. Professor Xu is a well-respected expert on the use of Qigong for medical purposes. He has worked at the highest levels of the Chinese government. One of his special gifts is the ability to understand meridians and meridian blockages from an energy or Qi standpoint, and the medical problems to which they are related.

Wu Ming Meridian Therapy is based on the ancient meridian theory that is described in Chapter 6. Remember, as we have emphasized many times throughout this book, when your organs function in harmony and Qi flows freely or unobstructed through your meridians, it is not possible to get cancer or any other illness or disease. And, even if you have had cancer, as long as you work toward this state, you have the ability to prevent cancer's return.

Wu Ming Meridian Therapy is designed to help your organs function in harmony and increase overall Qi. Each movement targets a specific meridian that runs through the breast area so you can unblock stagnating Qi and restore its free flow. Our energy movements are not physical exercises. You can think of them as meridian stretches or meridian therapy. They can also help you recall your own healing ability so you can help yourself.

Understanding the importance of the "healing message" behind *Wu Ming* Meridian Therapy is like understanding the performance of a great musician. While this musician might be able to teach his or her best students techniques for making beautiful music, he or she can only pass along the spirit or soul of the performance. This part can't be taught, but it can be known. In TCM, the best healing knowledge is passed similarly from master to student—often over the course of centuries and even millennia. In a similar way, I am passing you a healing message with the energy movements of *Wu Ming* Meridian Therapy. Following my instructions for the movements can convey to you many healing benefits. Through continual practice, you will have many opportunities to receive the strong healing message behind *Wu Ming* Meridian Therapy.

The following remarks by one of my patients and students talk about the benefits of this ancient practice:

"I saw something recently that really inspired me. It also mirrored for me my feelings about Qigong. During the broadcast of the Olympic games, a men's figure skating champion missed the gold medal and won the silver. In his postperformance interview, he told of how he skated in this important event with a painful groin injury and the after-effects of the flu. When asked if he was disappointed with his performance, he responded that he gave his 100 percent best considering his physical state. Gaining such remarkable strength, trusting in yourself and having courage to be your best, no matter what, is also the essence of my experience of Qigong.

As a mother and designer, I am looking forward to completing many projects as I near retirement age. Three years ago after being diagnosed with kidney cancer as well as an incurable blood disorder, I underwent a painful operation. My kidney and adrenal gland were removed to stop my cancer's spread. With less than a 30 percent five-year survival to look forward to, I soon realized that my doctors could no longer help me. Then I discovered Qigong, specifically *Wu Ming* Meridian Therapy, taught by Dr. Nan Lu. (We students also call him Master Lu.) Today, after more than three years of this training, the cancer and blood disorder are in control and my doctors befuddled.

What this amazing self-healing system did for me was help develop my inner strength, which in turn helped improve my physical condition and mental state. It returned me to myself. Although I came to Qigong almost out of desperation, I immediately sensed its power and that it would enable me to improve my life, ill or not. This form of Qi or energy training is true development at the highest level.

As a student and patient of Dr. Lu, I also undergo acupuncture treatments and take classical Chinese herbs as a complement to *Wu Ming* Qigong. Daily practice, weekly group practice, herbs and acupuncture are essential for me at this time. I intend to continue Qigong as an integral part of life. Like the figure skating champion, I also intend to give life 100 percent my best, whatever my limitations. I know deep in my heart that *Wu Ming* Meridian Therapy will help me do this."

If you use our companion video to help you practice *Wu Ming* Meridian Therapy, you can gain additional benefits by matching with the frequencies that are in it. The video has two parts: The first part reviews the whole movement and important details about it; the second allows you to follow me through the complete set of *Wu Ming* Meridian Therapy movements in real time, which takes about twenty minutes.

I recommend that you practice the full set of seven movements daily. As your practice develops, you will gradually help unblock stagnating Qi and begin to experience many health benefits from these ancient self-healing movements. If you cannot practice every day, try your best to incorporate as many movements as possible into your daily routine. Remember, this is your opportunity to take control of your own health and healing. The results can be remarkable. Here are some simple guidelines.

1. Always practice in comfortable clothing.

2. The entire program of seven movements should only take about twenty minutes a day. Try to practice at least once a day and at the same time. A good time to increase Qi is from 11:00 A.M. to 1:00 P.M. and from 5:00 P.M. to 7:00 P.M. It's also good to practice during the full moon, as well as during seasonal transitions like the winter solstice, spring equinox, and so on. Your birthday and birth time and your parents' birthdays are also especially good times to practice.

3. Besides practicing the entire set together, I recommend you practice each movement individually whenever you can. For maximum benefit, you must practice a movement at least five minutes, when you perform them separately. Even if you can't practice the entire set at one time, try to use any available minutes to perform any one of these movements. Also, the last movement is designed to build harmony among your organs and help strengthen the foundation of your kidney Qi. Try to hold this posture for as long as possible; the longer the better. If you practice long enough, you can reach a state where your mind will shut itself off and your body, mind, and spirit will become one.

4. Breathe naturally. *Wu Ming* Meridian Therapy requires no special breathing techniques.

5. There is no special mental focus. Try to remain peaceful and concentrate on what you are doing. Before practice try some deep breathing and give yourself an overall positive message of self-healing. Do not focus on a particular organ or meridian. If your mind cannot remain peaceful, then try to focus on the thought that you are receiving natural healing energy from the sun, the moon, the stars, and the entire Universe. At the same time, imagine that this natural healing energy is filling your body and destroying all cancer and illness. See yourself becoming healthier and healthier. Do not focus on a particular organ or body part.

6. When you reach a certain level in this ancient self-healing Qigong system, you will notice that the Qigong energy itself will cut off your thoughts and help you enter a timeless space where you can access your own self-healing power.

7. Do not practice when you are very hungry, after a big meal, if you are very tired, or after sex.

8. These are not aerobic or physical exercises. They are very gentle meridian stretches. Do each movement slowly.

Following are descriptions of the seven *Wu Ming* Meridian Therapy movements. Though they appear to be simple, they are very powerful energy movements that can make a big difference in the way you feel. These are lifelong healing gifts that spring from a very special ancient lineage. This is the most important self-healing information I can share with you.

1. THE DRAGON OPENS THE CURTAINS

Helps Relieve Qi Stagnation in the Upper Body

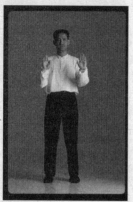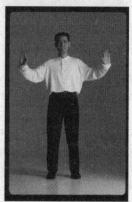

Stand with your feet shoulder wide. Raise your arms to shoulder level. Drop your elbows down. Bring your arms back at chest level. Keep your palms facing forward. Move hands in and out slowly at the same time. Each movement in and out counts as one. Do this for a total of two minutes.

2. THE DRAGON TOUCHES THE MOON

Lung Meridian (p. 249, top)

Stand with your feet shoulder wide and raise your arms to shoulder level. Drop your elbows down. Bring your arms back at chest level. Keep your palms facing forward. Push your hands forward slightly and bring them back. In this exercise, your arms should never fully straighten out. Always keep them bent. Each movement out and back counts as one. Do this for a total of two minutes.

The first two movements help Qi flow more freely through the entire breast and are particularly good for relieving breast tenderness.

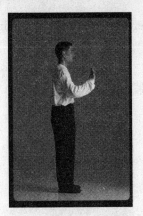
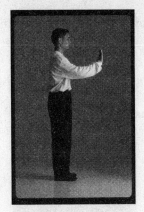

3. THE DRAGON'S TOE DANCE

Liver Meridian

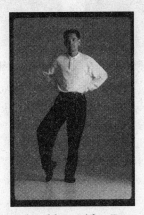

Stand with your feet shoulder wide. Put your hands on your waist. Put your weight on your right side. Raise your left heel and keep your left toe on the floor. Make a circle outward with your toe stationary on the floor, making sure your ankle, knee, and hip joints turn together at the same time. Each circle counts as one. Do this side for at least one minute.

Now, shift your weight to your left side. Raise your right heel and keep your right toe on the floor. Make a circle outward with your toe stationary on the floor. Make sure your ankle, knee, and hip joints turn together at the same time. Each circle counts as one. Do this side for at least one minute.

4. THE DRAGON KICKS FORWARD

Stomach Meridian

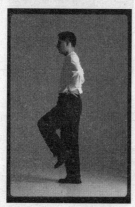 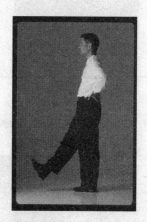

Stand with your feet shoulder wide. Put your hands at your waist. Start with your left leg. Bend your knee first then kick straight forward leading with your heel. Let your whole leg stretch out. Do not kick fast or high. Remember to stand straight. Each kick forward counts as one. Stop and change to your right leg. Do each side for at least one minute.

5. THE DRAGON KICKS BACKWARD

Bladder and Kidney Meridians (p. 251, top)
Stand with your feet shoulder wide. Put your hands at your waist. Start with your left leg. Bend your knee first then kick straight back with your heel. Make sure your leg is stretched out and that you do not kick too fast or too high. Each kick backward counts as one. Stop and change to the right leg. Do each side for at least one minute.

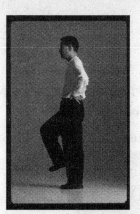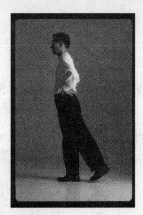

6. THE DRAGON SCOOPS THE MOON FROM THE OCEAN

Spleen and Stomach Meridians

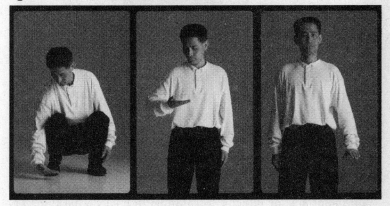

Stand with your feet shoulder wide. Bend with your knees slowly. Scoop with your left hand with palm facing upward. Stand up and raise your palm to chest level at the same time. Your palm is still facing up. Now, turn your palm and slowly drop your arm down at your side. Bend with your knees and scoop with your right hand with palm facing upward. Stand up and raise your palm to chest level at the same time. Your palm is still facing up. Turn your palm and slowly drop your arm down at your side. Do each side for two minutes.

7. THE DRAGON STANDS BETWEEN HEAVEN AND EARTH

Kidney Meridian and Harmonizing All Meridians

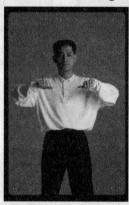

Stand with your feet shoulder wide. Bend your knees slightly. Make a fist and point your thumbs toward each other at chest level. Relax your shoulders. Close your eyes and imagine you are the Dragon standing between heaven and earth. Feel this power. Hold this special energy posture for at least three minutes. The longer you can hold it the better. An increase in your Qi comes only at the last few moments when it seems uncomfortable or difficult to continue to hold the posture. Try to push through this feeling. Eventually you will come to love this posture. You will want to stay in this position as long as possible. Many patients come back to tell me this. They even say that they don't want to answer the phone, or talk to anyone, or be interrupted in any way while practicing!

Open your eyes slowly and keep this special feeling. Remember that these ancient secrets of energy healing can help you prevent breast cancer or its recurrence. *Wu Ming* Meridian Therapy is one kind of Taoist Qi practice. To gain maximum benefit from this ancient energy healing art, you should simply be with this healing energy. The principle of this practice is that "no technique is the best technique." So remember—our meridian therapy demands no special concentration, no special breathing, no visualizations, no mind focus. The Qi you're building should be gentle, joyful, peaceful, and calm.

CHAPTER 17

Foods and Herbs You Can Use to Strengthen Your Healing Energy

Food is better than herbs,
Qi is better than food, and
Emptiness is better than Qi.

—*Traditional Taoist Maxim*

ONE major TCM principle we've discussed is that each individual is a part of the greater Universe. When you are born, you receive the Qi of both heaven and earth; you also receive both invisible and visible gifts. Thousands of years ago, healers in China understood this concept and saw that the human body, mind, and spirit are a unified whole with inseparable ties to nature. They also saw how the body's organs and systems interact with each other and change at the level of energy, or Qi. Modern physics is now recognizing this concept of dynamic patterns which interact, change, and transform on the level of energy thousands of years after it was solidly in place as part of TCM theory.

THE BODY RESPONDS TO NATURAL FORMS OF HEALING

TCM's First Focus is on Prevention

According to the traditional Taoist saying above, food is considered better than herbs for maintaining a healthy body. This phrase supports one of TCM's essential principles—prevention. We've already talked about one of the longstanding ways TCM has been practiced, where the doctor was paid only if his or her patient remained well. Focus on daily lifestyle and prevention has always been one of the strongest practices of TCM. This means that what you do on a daily basis can create many cumulative health benefits; conversely, daily negative habits can destroy your health. We don't really have this philosophy in the West. Most people become ill and then try to find someone to fix their problem. There is very little real focus on daily lifestyle choices. Basically the *Tao Te Ching* reminds us with the saying above that when it comes to eating, what you put into your body every day has a far greater effect on your overall health than an occasional visit to the doctor for herbs when you're sick.

One popular Chinese expression characterizes the wrong approach to eating: "You eat for your mouth and someone else's stomach!" Ideally, you should use your intuition to select foods and not rely on the desires of your eyes or tongue. As your body's Qi becomes stronger and more balanced, you will see that your body itself will guide this process, not your mind. Once again women with breast cancer can help themselves tremendously by applying this ancient healing knowledge. In the meantime, here are a few guidelines for mapping out an intelligent approach for eating:

🍃 A varied diet consisting primarily of vegetables, fruits, beans, nuts, and some grains, helps to keep your body in balance and its Qi flowing smoothly.

🍃 Seafood, particularly shellfish, has many healing benefits.

🍃 Large quantities of meat tend to put a burden on your digestive system and demand excess Qi to process. Try to avoid eating too much meat.

🍃 Certain Chinese herbs provide significant healing benefits to help prevent cancer or help strengthen the immune system during cancer treatments and can be included in your daily diet as foods. I've added some very good recipes in the following section that use herbs in combination with foods or are used as foods themselves. Scientific studies are now proving the efficacy of a number of Chinese herbs that have been in use for thousands of years.

HOW YOU EAT IS ALSO IMPORTANT

Not only what you eat but how you eat can greatly affect your overall health. These simple guidelines can also help make your self-healing program more successful:

🍃 Eating the greatest quantity of food earlier in the day allows your body to fully use its nutrition when it's needed the most.

🍃 Eating earlier in the evening and not late at night gives your digestive organs a rest while your body is sleeping, again saving more Qi for healing.

🍃 Eating "softly" (maintaining a quiet and relaxed manner while eating) helps make your digestive process easier.

🍃 Chewing your food thoroughly also helps to make digestion easier.

🐦 Stopping eating when you're about 70 percent full ensures that you do not force your digestive organs to use excess Qi.

Most of us tend to want big miracles in our lives. Small efforts like these done on a daily basis promote good health and help conserve your Qi or vital energy, which can better be accumulated for self-healing.

TCM Tip for Self-Healing

🐦 In general, native foods that are plentiful in a given season are the best to eat.

FOLLOW THE SEASONS

One of the most powerful things we can do for ourselves is to eat for health, not just for survival. This is done by following nature and the natural law. Ideally, your diet should follow the seasons. How do you know which food is right for which season? This is a particularly difficult question to answer when our grocery stores are full of fruits and vegetables from around the world or offer produce grown in greenhouses. The answer is that in general, native foods that are plentiful in a given season are the best to eat.

For instance, summer is the heart's season because summer's energy and weather can directly affect this organ's Qi as well as its function. A special healing fruit that is plentiful in America in the summer is watermelon. This is an ideal food with the unique ability to relieve summer's heat as well as the body's internal heat. Fall is the lung's season. A lot of people catch a cough at this time. Some fruits that are plentiful in the fall are pears and persimmons. They have a special, unique ability to relieve the dryness of the coughs of this particular season and strengthen lung Qi. How did TCM come to understand the healing benefits of foods and their specific relationship to the organs and meridians? Specially trained TCM doctors with the ability to "see" the actual Qi or essence of a food and how it relates to particular organs and meridians passed this knowledge down for generations from master to student until eventually it was captured in medical textbooks. Today, there are still a few masters that have this gift. I have been fortunate enough to study with them and receive some of this knowledge.

NATURAL PREFERENCES

According to TCM theory, each internal organ has a natural energy "preference." The liver prefers energy that flows smoothly. The spleen "likes" dryness and hates dampness while its partner the stomach likes all warm energies and can't stand cold energy. It is important to keep this in mind, especially when eating. Interestingly, the TCM doctor uses these natural energy preferences to help identify health problems, rebalance certain conditions or prevent them. For example, I often surprise my patients and students by telling them to avoid eating uncooked or raw foods. These things have a cold essence and, eaten frequently, can cause a stomach and spleen Qi deficiency. Even though raw foods may have a little more vitamins and nutrition than cooked foods, you will expend much more Qi in the chore of digestion. For women with breast cancer or those who want to prevent a recurrence, this is Qi you should be banking for self-healing.

To illustrate this: I had a patient come to me for stomach problems. He could never be in a group because he was constantly embarrassed by the loud gurgling sounds his stomach made and the fact that he constantly passed gas. He often suffered from stomach distention and stomach pain. This condition had become so bad that it had ruined his personal life. By the time I saw him, he had visited many doctors and was desperate. None of his doctors were able to help his condition. My classical diagnosis was that he was suffering from a liver and stomach function disorder. In other words, these two organs, so vital for good health, could not work in harmony. After several weeks of acupuncture and herbal therapy, his stomach pain, burping, and distention disappeared. The only complaint that remained was his stomach gas. I was puzzled. Because he had such a tremendous improvement, I knew that my diagnosis was correct and the treatments appropriate, but his gas should have disappeared as well. We had already discussed avoiding cold foods such as ice cream and cold drinks such as soda. And, I didn't think to probe further about his eating habits. It turned out that I had missed one important thing. This man loved raw vegetables. Every day he ate large quantities of things like cauliflower, broccoli, and cold salads. Then I realized that we had uncovered the missing piece of the puzzle! I told him to stop eating raw vegetables and that everything he ate should be either steamed or cooked. I also advised him to add as much cinnamon and ginger as he could whenever he cooked. After changing his eating habits, this problem that had plagued him for so many years and literally made him a prisoner finally was cured. His whole life changed. As a native Chinese man and TCM doctor, I learned an important lesson. To tell you the truth, it never occurred to me that Americans would eat such large quantities of raw vegetables with the belief that they were doing the healthy thing.

ENERGY ESSENCE

All things in nature, food and herbs included, have a special signature essence, which is called an "energy essence." This attribute moves beyond tangible, measurable qualities such as nutritional value, calories, vitamins, ect. to describe invisible things like how something (in this case, a particular food or herb) affects certain internal organs, which meridians it travels to, and what impact it has on the body's overall Qi.

One way to understand the concept of essence is to look at how homeopathy works. It takes a substance and dilutes it many hundreds of times. At the point of maximum dilution, there is obviously not enough of the substance to physically affect the individual's health, but the essence or energy of the substance is still active. That is why the principle of homeopathy can help certain conditions.

Instead of diluting a substance, TCM focuses on concentrating several substances together. Sometimes it uses an individual herb; most of the time it uses a combination of herbs and concentrates these substances by cooking them, in many cases for hours at a time. Physically, all their properties have been rendered useless for nutrition or vitamin content. However, they still have the power to fix a health problem. Why? Because their energy essence still works. This helps us understand why cooking certain combinations of foods for a very long time still can provide healing benefits. TCM also perceives another type of essence called natural essence. In this concept, like things can fix like things. For example, the skin or bark of a tree may be used to fix skin problems. The roots of a tree may help problems deeply rooted within the body. Bones or bone marrow may be used to help restore health to the kidney or relieve bone (the tissue of the kidney) problems. That's why delicious bone marrow soup can actually help strengthen your bones better that taking calcium supplements.

CHINESE HERBS:
A TCM HEALING RESOURCE

While certain foods have medicinal value in addition to their nutritional properties, it is classical Chinese herbs that form a major TCM healing resource. TCM has thousands of years of study and practical experience in the use of herbs. In the West, herbs are often selected in accordance with symptoms, e.g., *dong qai* is beneficial for menstrual problems; ginseng is good for low energy. You can end up taking a large number of herbs at the same time based on the symptoms you're experiencing. As we have seen, the TCM understanding of herbs and herbal formulations, as well as their usage, is completely different.

In dealing with any health problem, TCM's first course of action is to look beyond symptoms to find the root cause. The whole focus with Chinese herbs is internal, not external. For instance, while the dolichos seed has many nutritive properties, a doctor of TCM would use it for its ability to effect a change in your spleen and stomach Qi or energies. The purpose of this treatment then is not on giving added nutrition, but rather on helping to maximize the way your internal organs function through the use of herbs. Using herbs this way goes beyond healing in the sense of "fixing." This is an "energy" approach to herbs—using their essences, or particular Qi to heal the internal organs. Interestingly enough, when your internal organs heal, you can gain maximum nutrition from a minimum amount of food. Here again your body is reaching a state where you can save more Qi for healing. This is so important if you have breast cancer or are trying to prevent a recurrence. The TCM goal also is to balance the energy relationships between the internal organs—helping them communicate better through Qi—so they function well and in harmony with each other. This creates the foundation for true healing and good health.

HOW CHINESE HERBAL FORMULAS WORK

Chinese herbs are sometimes used individually, but most often they are used in a formula or combination of herbs. Formulas are made to work on the underlying cause (or causes) of a health problem. These formulas must also take into account who they are prepared for, where that person lives, and when they will be taken.

For example, "China Dirt," an herbal compound I use in my practice for patients with weight problems, is specifically formulated for Western people who generally suffer from stomach and liver function problems. Because of the stressful lives they lead, these people's organs, while physically normal, usually do not work properly, either alone or in partnership with their other organs. This is actually the root cause of their weight problems. "China Dirt" contains dolichos seed, Chinese yam, and lotus seed—all of which increase the Qi of the stomach and spleen and help the stomach function very well. This herbal combination also has coix seed and orange peel. These two herbs, in addition to being cancer preventatives, relieve internal dampness (which tends to impair the digestive function) and coordinate digestive function. Corn silk is added to guide the Qi of these herbs to the liver and gallbladder, while hawthorn berries increase metabolism, process fat and water, as well as decrease fat and the level of cholesterol. The overall goal of this herbal formula is to help the entire digestive system of a Western individual function better.

The key dynamic of this formula and the TCM approach to using herbs in combination is that they're designed to work as a team. Each herb has an individual role that supports the overall purpose of the formula. Changing just one herb—either adding it, removing it, or changing the amount—alters the entire formula. There is an analogy I use when explaining the difference between the Eastern and Western approach to herbs. I tell my patients and students that TCM uses herbs the way a coach assembles a first-rate football team; the typical Western approach is more like working with a single athlete (for example a tennis player or a golfer).

THE PURPOSE OF HERBS AND TCM FOR BREAST CANCER

For thousands of years, TCM has studied from experience a number of herbs that are beneficial for treating the underlying internal conditions for what we in the West term breast cancer. TCM has also had extensive experience with using herbs for breast problems that are early warning signs of breast cancer. Herbs (many of them are actually foods but are used traditionally in an herbal context) such as dolichos seed, coix seed, red sage root, psoralea fruit, and tangerine peel have been included in these herbal formulas for centuries. The purpose of the herbs available through my Breast Cancer Prevention Project is to help the liver, stomach, and kidney function properly. When these three organs, whose meridians run through 80 percent of the areas where breast cancer occurs, work in harmony, TCM believes that conditions for breast cancer can be almost completely controlled.

As we've seen, TCM believes breast cancer develops because these organs and their meridians are experiencing a dysfunction. Often, an organ's function is off balance for many years before any organic or physical problem develops in that organ or can be detected in any scientific test. In light of this, it's interesting to note that Western doctors theorize that most breast cancers have been in place about eight to ten years before they're detected.

Let's review these three key organs again and then look at the special list of healing foods and herbs that TCM includes in an "eating for healing" plan. I've adapted these foods from a much broader list to suit Western preferences. For the most part, you'll be surprised at the everyday foods that TCM prescribes to help patients recapture their good health. I've also listed many herbs that TCM practitioners have used for centuries to heal these three very important organs.

❧What Is the Liver's Function?

According to TCM, the liver's function is to keep internal Qi and blood moving freely throughout the body. The liver's job is also to remove stagnant Qi wherever it occurs. This is extremely important for women, since TCM sees stagnation of Qi and/or blood as a causative factor in the development of masses or tumors. Because both the liver and stomach meridians travel through the breast area, the free flow of energy through them, as well as the proper functioning of the liver, become crucial for breast health.

❧How Does the Stomach Function?

The liver controls the stomach, according to TCM theory, and any irregularity in the liver's Qi will naturally affect the function of the stomach. The liver's responsibility for regulating the smooth flow of Qi also extends to help the stomach and spleen perform their digestive functions. TCM considers the stomach (and spleen) the material source of Qi and blood in the body. If they are not functioning properly, the health of the whole body is affected. Fifty percent of breast cancers occur in the area through which the stomach meridian runs.

❧Why Is Kidney Function Important?

In TCM's view, the kidney is of critical importance because it is the main source of Qi for the entire body. This is an inherited source of Qi which comes from our parents. Kidney Qi declines naturally with age. The TCM herbs in our Breast Cancer Prevention Project help to support and strengthen the kidney Qi, so that it can function at a higher level for a longer time. These three organs—the liver, the stomach and the kidney—comprise a unique triangular closed system with tremendous feedback capacity that uniquely reflects Western health problems. Stress and emotional problems directly affect your liver; Western diet directly causes stomach problems, and the Western lifestyle of constant work and motion directly affects the kidney. In my experience, concentrating on treating this "closed end system" produces the greatest health benefits for my Western patients.

WHO MAKES THE HERBAL FORMULA IS A KEY POINT

While the formula itself is important, of equal importance in traditional Chinese medicine is the person who makes and dispenses it. The depth of understanding and level of Qi of the doctor or herbalist are key to how well the treatment works. The following story about a doctor in the Qing dynasty illustrates this point very well.

The Falling Leaf

Hundreds of years ago, the wife of a powerful king was expecting a baby. Although this was a joyful occasion, there was much concern for the queen because her delivery was quite delayed. The king feared for his wife and his unborn child. Many famous doctors were called to the kingdom to help. One by one, each doctor prescribed herbs but nothing seemed to work.

One day, a wise and very esteemed doctor who possessed great understanding of the ways of the Universe came to the kingdom. On the day of the autumnal equinox, he attended the queen and checked the herbs she had been given. Just at that very moment, a leaf fell from a tree overhead. The doctor caught the leaf and added it to his herbal mixture saying, "Now it is perfect. Drink the herbs and all will be well." Shortly thereafter, the queen gave birth to her child.

This doctor had a deep understanding of the principles of Universal energy and knew how to apply this knowledge in practice. His consultation with the queen had taken place on the day of the autumnal equinox. On this day, the energy of the seasons begins to turn—summer becomes fall. The leaf, following this shift in energy, fell from the tree at the perfect moment. The doctor knew that the leaf had received the "energy message" from the Universe of letting go and that the leaf could be used as a communications vehicle to bring this same energy essence into the Queen's body. And so the birth took place, because the baby now also knew it was the correct time to let go. In the hands of a skilled and high-level practitioner, herbs (and other healing techniques) can ultimately transfer healing Qi.

TCM BUILDS HEALTH FROM THE INSIDE OUT

Before proceeding to the Food Section, let's return once more to our Taoist maxim: "Qi is better than food or herbs." It is important to understand this concept and let you understand that Qi is a powerful and effective way to build health from the inside out. As we reviewed earlier, the self-healing practice of Chinese Qigong is thousands of years old. Through simple movements and postures, it helps to balance the body's internal Qi and raise it to a higher level. If your internal Qi is strong and flowing smoothly, your body is healthy. It functions well as a whole so you can absorb and create energy from the foods you eat.

And how is "emptiness," a very important ancient TCM principle, better than all the rest? "Nothing is everything," as one famous traditional Taoist saying puts it. Since its beginnings, TCM has recognized the strong role the emotions, the mind, and the spirit play in health. It is possible to eat a nutritious diet and practice Qigong hours and hours every day, but if your mind is disturbed and your spirit is not peaceful, attempts to build and conserve Qi are hindered. When we're empty, or without judgment, we're one with the Tao; we are in harmony with the way of the everchanging Universe. There is no resistance, we live in a relaxed and completely open and flowing way. The Universe has its own way to achieve balance, and as a mirror of the greater whole, we also have an inborn balancing or healing ability. Remember your own powerful self-healing mechanism is able to fully emerge when you are truly empty. In this sense, emptiness is the most powerful healing technique of all.

HEALING FOODS FOR BREAST CANCER PREVENTION AND TREATMENT

Broccoli

ESSENCE: Neutral

MERIDIANS: Enters the heart and large intestine meridians

EFFECTS:

- Benefits the heart and liver; specifically, it decreases internal heat in these two organs
- Helps prevent heart disease

NOTES: Sauté, steam, or juice

Cauliflower

ESSENCE: Neutral

MERIDIANS: Enters the large intestine and kidney meridians

EFFECTS:

- Increases kidney Qi
- Helps gallbladder infection
- Good for constipation

Scallion

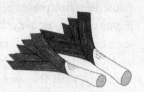

ESSENCE: Warm

MERIDIANS: Enters the stomach and liver meridians

EFFECTS:

- Benefits the stomach and liver
- Relieves body of internal cold conditions (i.e., cold in the stomach, liver, and lung)
- Helps menstrual difficulties (PMS, painful periods, irregular periods, etc.)
- Helps headaches, colds
- Relieves skin rashes and infections

NOTES: The following recipes use scallions to promote healing.

PMS Tea

INGREDIENTS:

4 pieces of ginger

3 whole scallions

Peel from 1 orange

1 handful of dried rose petals (buy yourself a dozen roses and dry the blooms!)

1 pinch of rosemary

1 pinch of cinnamon

DIRECTIONS:

Place all ingredients in a pot of water (about 2 quarts) and let the tea steep; drink hot, two times per day while symptoms are present.

Relief for Lower Stomach Pain, Difficulty Urinating, and PMS

INGREDIENTS:
   1–2 scallions, chopped or smashed
   2–3 tablespoons of wine or vinegar

DIRECTIONS:
   Put ingredients in a wok and heat; put mixture in cheese-cloth or toweling and apply to lower stomach as a compress.

For Colds with Headache, Runny Nose, and Chills

INGREDIENTS:
   5–10 scallions, the white part only
   2 pieces of ginger
   brown sugar

DIRECTIONS:
   Add scallions and ginger to water in a pot and bring to a boil; add brown sugar and drink hot.

For Skin Rashes, Itching, and Infection

   Use the white part only of 5–10 scallions; smash, add honey to make a paste, and apply to the skin; this mixture helps relieve itching and infection.

Ginger

ALTERNATE ENGLISH NAMES: None
LATIN NAME: *Rhizoma zingiberis*
PINYIN: Jiang
FLAVOR: Pungent
ESSENCE: Warm
MERIDIANS: Enters the stomach, heart, and
   lung meridians

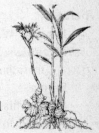

EFFECTS:

- Benefits the digestive organs, particularly the stomach
- Relieves digestive problems
- Gets rid of internal cold conditions
- Warms the lung
- Helps liver Qi to flow smoothly (relieves blockages in the liver)
- Cancer (preventive)

INDICATIONS:

- Digestive problems such as nausea, loose stool, cold in the stomach, stomach infections, food poisoning
- Lung difficulties, especially associated with cold (cough, shortness of breath, retention of phlegm)
- Menstrual difficulties (PMS, cramping)
- Sports injuries

DOSAGE: 3–10 grams, decocted in water for an oral dose

NOTES: Fresh ginger is particularly good for the lung; for sports injuries, rub fresh ginger over the affected area (peel off the skin first).

PMS Compress

Make a mixture of equal amounts of fennel, cayenne pepper, and grated fresh ginger to equal ½ lb. (8 oz.); steam or bake in the oven until very warm; place mixture in a clean cotton cloth and apply to painful area on abdomen until the warmth dissipates.

Fennel

ESSENCE: Warm

MERIDIANS: Enters the liver, kidney, spleen, and stomach meridians

EFFECTS:

- Benefits the liver and the stomach
- Good for stomachache caused by internal cold

- Relieves food poisoning
- Helps to regulate menstrual cycle, relieves PMS

Garlic

ESSENCE: Warm

MERIDIANS: Enters the stomach and large intestine meridians

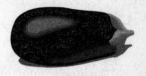

EFFECTS:

- Benefits the liver and stomach
- Helpful for stomachache caused by internal cold
- Relieves food poisoning
- Good for general body pain

Eggplant

ESSENCE: Neutral

MERIDIANS: Enters the liver, large intestine, and urinary bladder meridians

EFFECTS:

- Helps balance liver function, relieves liver problems
- Beneficial for weight loss
- Protects against high cholesterol
- Relieves coughs
- Helps the condition of hepatitis

Celery

ESSENCE: Warm

MERIDIANS: Enters the spleen and stomach meridians

EFFECTS:

- Increases stomach Qi
- Relieves joint pain
- Promotes sleep (useful for insomnia)
- Good for high blood pressure and diabetes

NOTES: Celery juice is very beneficial; include celery in soups and other vegetable recipes.

Carrot

ESSENCE: Cold

MERIDIANS: Enters the stomach and spleen meridians

EFFECTS:

- Relieves cough and conditions of mucus in the lung, good for asthma
- Beneficial for stomach problems

NOTES: To get the benefit of vitamin A from carrots, they must be cooked with some oil.

Chinese Pear

ESSENCE: Cold

MERIDIANS: Enters the lung and large intestine meridians

EFFECTS:

- Greatly benefits the lung, relieves heat in the lung, especially during radiation and chemotherapy

NOTES: Freshly squeezed pear juice helps the lung; following is a Chinese recipe for pears.

Traditional Cooked Pears

INGREDIENTS:

6 pears, chopped

1/3 cup rock sugar candy (available at Chinese food stores)

1/4 cup water

DIRECTIONS:

Place all ingredients in a 2–quart covered pot and double boil on low to medium heat for approximately 40 minutes (for those not familiar with the method of double boiling, place the covered pot containing the pears in another pot with several inches of water in it; the larger outside pot is the one that comes into contact with the heat source).

Kiwi

ESSENCE: Cold

MERIDIANS: Enters the lung, large intestine, and stomach meridians

EFFECTS:

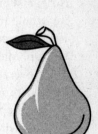

- Benefits the lung, good for lung infections, relieves cough and heat in the lung
- Helps relieve the side effects of radiation and chemotherapy, reduces internal heat in the lung and stomach

American Pear

ESSENCE: Cold

MERIDIANS: Enters the large intestine and lung meridians

EFFECTS:

- Greatly benefits the lung, relieves heat in the lung, especially during radiation and chemotherapy

NOTES: Freshly squeezed pear juice helps the lung. American Pears can be used in the same recipe above for Chinese Pears.

Lemon

ESSENCE: Warm

MERIDIANS: Enters the large intestine and kidney meridians

EFFECTS:

- Helps increase kidney energy
- Diuretic; relieves edema

Watermelon

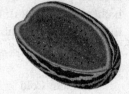

ESSENCE: Cold

MERIDIANS: Enters the liver, heart, urinary bladder, and stomach meridians

EFFECTS:

- Relieves thirst
- Decreases internal heat
- Increases the frequency of urination
- Releases toxins from the body
- Beneficial in the treatment of kidney infections
- Helps liver disease
- Beneficial for heart problems, high blood pressure
- Helps the condition of diabetes

NOTES: When juicing watermelon, be sure and use the whole fruit, especially the green and white of the rind. Watermelon is also excellent for overexposure to the sun. Make a juice from the whole watermelon and wash it over the skin. This will help to cool the skin down and promote healing. Many people in the West throw out the most valuable part of the watermelon, the rind. Following is a Chinese recipe for watermelon rind.

Cooked Watermelon Rinds

INGREDIENTS:

2 cups of watermelon rind cut into 1-inch cubes (cut off green skin but leave a little red on rind for color)

1 teaspoon soy sauce

1/2 teaspoon sliced ginger

1 teaspoon sugar

3 or 4 chopped scallions (separate white and green parts)

2 teaspoons corn oil

Pinch of salt

DIRECTIONS:

Preheat wok on medium-high heat and add corn oil; add white part of scallions and cook for a few minutes, adding the pinch of salt; add watermelon cubes and sliced ginger and stir-fry until a little water comes out of the watermelon; add soy sauce, sugar, and green part of scallions, stir well.

Red and White (Daikon) Radish

ESSENCE: Neutral

MERIDIANS: Enters the lung and stomach
meridians

EFFECTS:

- Relieves heat in the lung
- Breaks up stagnation of Qi and blood
- Helps coughs
- Beneficial for the digestive system (particularly good for stomach distention)

Pineapple

ESSENCE: Warm

MERIDIANS: Enters the small intestine and stomach meridians

EFFECTS:

- Helps PMS
- Beneficial for the digestive system (particularly helpful for loose stool)
- Relieves body of internal cold condition

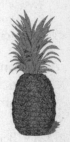

Chinese Red Date

ALTERNATE ENGLISH NAMES: Chinese date, jujube

LATIN NAME: *Fructus Zizyphi*

PINYIN: Hong zao

FLAVOR: Sweet

ESSENCE: Warm

MERIDIANS: Enters the spleen and stomach meridians

EFFECTS:

- Helps strengthen function of spleen and stomach
- Beneficial for the heart
- Strengthens overall Qi
- Restores lost body fluids
- Relieves depression, stabilizes mood swings

INDICATIONS:

- Digestive problems (such as poor appetite)
- Low energy, fatigue
- Excessive sweating, conditions where a large loss of body fluids has occurred
- Palpitations, racing of the heart
- Depression, especially that associated with PMS

DOSAGE: 10–15 grams, decocted in water for an oral dose

NOTES: Red dates can also be incorporated into vegetable recipes in addition to being used in a traditional herbal formula; the Chinese use red dates in a traditional-style porridge, eaten in the morning; add a small handful to your hot cereal, favorite vegetarian soup, or cooked rice. Eat as often as possible.

American Date

ESSENCE: Warm

MERIDIANS: Enters the spleen and stomach meridians

EFFECTS:

- Benefits the lung and stomach

NOTES: American dates are similar to Chinese red dates in essence but have less power.

Bamboo Shoots and Tips

ESSENCE: Neutral

MERIDIANS: Enters the stomach, small intestine, and spleen meridians

EFFECTS:
- Good for stagnation in the digestive system, poor appetite, weight problems, high cholesterol
- Helps prevent heart disease

Peanut

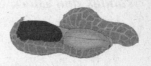

ESSENCE: Warm

MERIDIANS: Enters the kidney, stomach, spleen, and large intestine meridians

EFFECTS:
- Good for stomach and spleen (helps condition of loose stool)
- Increases T cells
- Helps to strengthen lung function

Chestnut

ESSENCE: Warm

MERIDIANS: Enters the stomach, spleen, and kidney meridians

EFFECTS:
- Strengthens both the stomach and kidney

Pine Nut

ESSENCE: Warm

MERIDIANS: Enters the kidney and lung meridians

EFFECTS:
- Beneficial for the kidney
- Helps constipation

Walnut

ESSENCE: Warm

MERIDIANS: Enters the kidney, lung, and large intestine meridians

EFFECTS:
- Beneficial for the kidney
- Helps constipation

Walnuts and Black Sesame Seeds

INGREDIENTS:
  $1/2$ *lb. walnuts*
  $1/2$ *lb. black sesame seeds*
  3 to 4 ounces honey

DIRECTIONS:

Grind ingredients together in a blender. Cook in a double boiler or steam for one hour. After cooking, refrigerate. Eat two tablespoons in the morning and two in the evening. This is a simple, yet delicious, recipe that can help strengthen and increase Qi. This recipe is especially good for longevity and maintaining healthy skin and hair. It can also help older people who suffer from constipation and cough.

Aduki Bean

LATIN NAME: *Phaseolus calcaratus (Roxb.)*
PINYIN: Chi xiao don
FLAVOR: Sweet and sour
ESSENCE: Neutral
MERIDIANS: Enters the heart and small intestine meridians
EFFECTS:
- Greatly benefits the kidney, relieves the body of excess water, decreases swelling
- Helps fight infections
- Relieves the body of toxins, poisons

INDICATIONS:
- Edema, particularly in the legs, knees, ankles; any condition of swelling

- Kidney and liver infections (which may be causing edema)
- Any kind of poison or infection (for example, skin infection)
- Breast masses and/or tumors

DOSAGE: As an "herb," 10–30 grams, decocted in water for an oral dose

NOTES: Aduki beans can also be cooked and eaten as a main or side dish: rinse beans and combine 1 cup of beans and 2–3 cups of water in a pot; bring to a boil, reduce heat and cook for approximately one hour or until soft; season with salt, pepper, and other herbs, such as parsley. As an external paste applied to skin infections: smash cooked beans and mix with honey, a small amount of vinegar (or use an egg white as a binding agent), and apply to skin.

Mung Bean

ESSENCE: Cold

MERIDIANS: Enters the heart, lung, and small intestine meridians

EFFECTS:

- Very beneficial for detoxifying conditions of infection (internal and external) in the body, skin problems, food poisoning
- Relieves internal heat, particularly in the liver and stomach

Black Bean

ESSENCE: Neutral

MERIDIANS: Enters the kidney and spleen meridians

EFFECTS:

- Very beneficial for the kidney
- Helps to regulate irregular menstruation

NOTES: Black beans are excellent as a soup: soak 2 cups overnight, combine with approximately 4 cups water, salt and pepper to taste, and a large handful of cilantro (also called "coriander" or "Chinese parsley") and bring to a boil, reduce heat and cook on low to medium heat for several hours until beans are soft.

Red Bean

PINYIN: Hung dou

ESSENCE: Neutral to slightly warm

MERIDIANS: Enters the stomach and spleen meridians

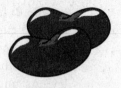

EFFECTS:

- Helps to strengthen and regulate the function of the stomach and spleen; improves the digestive system overall
- Increases T cells

Dandelion Greens

ALTERNATE ENGLISH NAMES: Priest's crown, swine's snout

LATIN NAME: *Herba Dens leonis*

PINYIN: Pu gong yin

FLAVOR: Bitter and sweet

ESSENCE: Cool

MERIDIANS: Enters the stomach, liver, and lung meridians

EFFECTS:

- Relieves internal heat in the body
- Detoxifies poisons, acts as a natural antibiotic
- Relieves conditions of internal dampness
- Tonic for the digestive system, particularly the liver and stomach

INDICATIONS:

- Skin problems/infections, sores
- Internal infections
- Breast area problems such as breast cancer, breast tumors and masses
- Digestive disturbances (which can be caused by conditions of excessive heat or dampness internally)

DOSAGE: 10–30 grams of dry powder taken in capsule or tea form for an oral dose

NOTES: Dandelion greens are nontoxic and larger doses are possible; if too much is eaten, they can cause loose stool (conversely, they can help constipation); dandelion greens can be sautéed, and used in soups. They can also be applied to skin sores and infections: smash the greens to a pulp and apply to the affected area (for example, to an infected or sore breast).

Lotus Seed

ALTERNATE ENGLISH NAME: Lotus nut

LATIN NAME: *Semen Nelumbinis*

PINYIN: Lian rou

FLAVOR: Astringent and sweet

ESSENCE: Neutral

MERIDIANS: Enters the spleen, kidney, and heart meridians

EFFECTS:

- Benefits the spleen, stomach, and lung
- Tones the digestive system (effective for symptoms of poor appetite, chronic diarrhea due to a deficiency of the spleen)
- Increases blood cells
- Strengthens the kidney
- Quiets the spirit

INDICATIONS:

- Digestive disturbances

- Conditions (such as after surgery) where there has been a large loss of blood (also, uterine bleeding)
- Insomnia, palpitations, restlessness

DOSAGE: 6–15 grams, decocted in water for an oral dose

    Precautions: Lotus seed should not be used in cases of constipation.

NOTES: Lotus root has all of the above-listed properties, but it is effective when used to stop bleeding; can be eaten raw, cooked, or juiced.

Mushroom

(Portobello, snowcap, fresh and dried shiitake, white fungus)

ESSENCE: Most have a neutral essence

MERIDIANS: Enters the stomach, spleen, and urinary bladder meridians

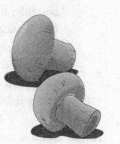

EFFECTS:

- Helps build the immune system
- Good for cancer prevention

NOTES: White fungus helps the lung and is good for coughs; additionally, it is good for sleeping problems.

Soy Products

Soy products such as soybeans, soybean curd (tofu), soy-milk, and soybean sprouts all are a good source of nutrition for the body.

MERIDIANS: Enters the kidney, stomach, and spleen meridians

ESSENCE OF THE SPROUTS: neutral to warm, they are the greatest source of nutrition.

NOTES: There are two styles of making bean curd or tofu; one creates a tofu with a cold essence, and the other (Japanese-style) creates a tofu with a warm to hot essence. If there is a condition of heat in the stomach, it is better to eat the former type (with a cold essence).

Honey with Honeycomb

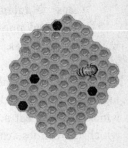

MERIDIANS: Enters the lung, large intestine, and spleen meridians

EFFECTS:
- Increases lung energy
- Moistens, helping constipation

NOTES: Honeycomb is very beneficial for arthritis pain.

Bee Pollen

MERIDIANS: Enters the heart, small intestine, lung, large intestine, and urinary bladder meridians

EFFECTS:
- Helps optimize the functioning of the immune system
- Beneficial for heart disease
- Helps to build the blood, increase blood circulation

NOTES: Bee pollen is one of the greatest of all natural foods; a spoonful can be eaten with juice every day.

Green Tea

ESSENCE: Cool (the caffeine in green tea is cool)

MERIDIANS: Enters the stomach and heart meridians

EFFECTS:
- Good for the blood
- Beneficial for the digestive system
- Decreases body fat

Seaweed

ESSENCE: Cool

MERIDIANS: Enters the liver, stomach, and kidney meridians

EFFECTS:
- Helps destroy masses and tumors
- Beneficial for thyroid problems

NOTES: There are many varieties of seaweed such as agar

agar (Kanten), arame, dulse, hijiki, Irish moss, kombu, and wakame. Seaweed can be added to soups and vegetable dishes.

You can buy the kind of seaweed that is used to make Japanese sushi. This kind of seaweed is also available as a snack, which you can eat anytime. There is another kind of seaweed, which the Chinese call *zi cai*. This seaweed is thicker than that used for sushi. You must cook this seaweed. You can combine the cooked seaweed with tomato and egg to create a delicious soup. There is an even thicker and wider seaweed, which the Chinese call *hai dai*. It can be bought dry and must be soaked before using. You can sauté *hai dai*, marinate it or make a soup with it.

Marinated Seaweed

INGREDIENTS:
2 pieces of thick dried seaweed
5 cloves of garlic
2 slices of fresh ginger
1 teaspoon of sesame oil
1 teaspoon of soy sauce
1 teaspoon of vinegar
pinch of salt and pepper
pinch of sugar

DIRECTIONS:
Rinse seaweed and soak it in water for about ten to fifteen minutes. Wash the seaweed and slice very finely. Boil a large pot of water. Put 1 teaspoon of salt in the water. Bring to boil. When the water boils, add the sliced seaweed. Bring to boil again. Then strain the water and rinse seaweed with cold water and strain again. Mince the garlic and ginger together. Then put

seaweed back in the pot, combine all of ingredients together. Mix well and refrigerate. You can eat this cold or at room temperature. Adjust to your taste with salt, pepper, sugar, and vinegar.

Chinese Barley

FLAVOR: Sweet
ESSENCE: Slightly cool
MERIDIANS: Enters the spleen, stomach, and lung meridians
EFFECTS:
- Relieves water and dampness in the body
- Strengthens the digestive system
- Relieves arthritis pain due to dampness
- Helps infections
- Helps to soften masses
- Cancer (preventive)

Sweet Barley and Red Date Soup

This recipe can help anyone strengthen their digestive system. It is a particularly good dish to eat during chemotherapy because it can help relieve some of its side effects, such as nausea, diarrhea, as well as lack of appetite.

Use 1 cup of Chinese barley with ½ cup of lotus seed and ½ cup each of red beans and Chinese red dates. Put all ingredients in one pot, cover with about 2 quarts of water. Bring to a boil; then cook down by simmering for about 1 hour until the beans and the barley open. Then add honey or sugar and cinnamon to taste. Eat hot for breakfast or at the end of a meal. NOTES: Chinese barley is similar to American barley but is more efficacious as a healing food; cook it for breakfast with water like porridge. Chinese barley can be bought at Chinese food stores.

Tangerine Peel

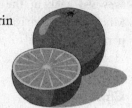

ALTERNATE ENGLISH NAMES: Mandarin peel, tangerine rind

LATIN NAME: *Pericarpium Citri reticulatae*

PINYIN: Chen pi

FLAVOR: Pungent and bitter

ESSENCE: Warm

MERIDIANS: Enters the stomach and lung meridians

EFFECTS:

- Balances the function of the spleen and stomach
- Balances Qi or vital energy
- Eliminates dampness in the stomach and upper abdominal area
- Clears up phlegm

INDICATIONS:

- Digestive problems involving abdominal distention, belching, nausea, vomiting, poor appetite, loose stool (these symptoms can be due to a stagnation of Qi in the spleen and stomach)
- Tiredness, fatigue
- Lung problems such as a full, "oppressed" feeling in the chest, cough, profuse sputum

DOSAGE: 3–10 grams, decocted in water for an oral dose

NOTES: Save tangerine rinds, let dry, and store for later use; you can grind the rinds to a powder to use; mix with honey and take as needed; the following recipe is very useful for coughs, excess mucous in the lungs, or sinus headache.

Tangerine Peel Tea

INGREDIENTS:
  2 *tangerine rinds*
  4 *scallions (each cut into 3 or 4 pieces)*
  1 *chunk ginger (leave skin on, smash whole)*
  A few almonds

DIRECTIONS:
  Put ingredients in water and bring to a boil, let mixture boil for only 2 to 4 minutes; add brown sugar or honey and drink. For a cold, take a hot bath, drink this mixture, go to bed, wrapping yourself up and sweat the cold out. For a scratchy throat, add a little peppermint to the mixture.

YOUR BREAST CANCER PREVENTION SHOPPING LIST

I recommend that you add these healing foods to your shopping list. Change your eating patterns to include as many of these as possible, as often as possible.

- Scallions, ginger, garlic, fennel

- Broccoli, cauliflower

- Eggplant, carrot, celery

- Radish, chinese radish

- Bamboo, lotus

- Beans, Chinese beans, Bean curd (tofu), bean sprouts, soy products (such as soy milk)

- Mushrooms (any kind)

- Nuts—walnuts, pine nuts, peanuts, chestnuts

- Dates

- Pineapples, watermelon

- Kiwi, lemon, pears

- Honey, bee pollen, honeycomb

- Barley

- All green teas—do not buy decaffeinated products

HEALING HERBS FOR BREAST CANCER PREVENTION AND TREATMENT

Following are a number of herbs used in TCM for breast cancer treatments. Many have been used for thousands of years. As with the food listed previously, I have selected those that are best for Western women. I have listed alternate English names of the herbs as well as their Latin and Pinyin names. (Pinyin is the system used to transform Chinese ideograms into words that can be pronounced.) Each of these entries also identifies the essence of the herb, the meridian or meridians it affects, as well as how it helps the body and which conditions it can improve. Dosages listed here are for average usage. When a condition changes, the TCM practitioner adjusts the dosage accordingly. This resource will provide you with deeper knowledge about TCM herbs that heal. It will help you work in partnership if you choose to complement Western breast cancer treatments by working with a TCM practitioner.

Remember we discussed earlier how TCM uses herbs. Most are used in the context of a team of herbs with each one assigned a specific role; some can be used singly or in small combinations. The Chinese pride themselves on being inventive and efficient. They like to kill two birds with one stone. So they have an entire portion of Chinese healing arts devoted to combining foods and herbs for the purpose of healing. This is known as *shi liao*, which means using food for healing purposes, or *yao shan*, which means using herbs as food to heal. Some herbs can be cooked together with other foods such as chicken, fish, pork or lamb to enhance their effects. A number of famous restaurants in China and Hong Kong serve meals of this kind. We've added a few ancient recipes at the end of this chapter that you can include in your own self-healing program.

Angelica Root

ALTERNATE ENGLISH NAMES: Dong quai, tangkuei root, Chinese angelica root

LATIN NAME: *Radix Angelicae sinensis*

PINYIN: Dang gui

FLAVOR: Sweet and pungent

ESSENCE: Warm

MERIDIANS: Enters the liver, heart, and spleen meridians

EFFECTS:

- Tones the blood (builds T cells), increases blood circulation
- Relieves pain
- Moistens the bowels
- Regulates menstruation

INDICATIONS:

- A condition of blood deficiency (such as that after surgery, cancer treatment; often manifesting with symptoms of pale lips and tongue, sallow complexion, dizziness, palpitations)
- Irregular menstruation (absence of periods, painful periods) uterine bleeding
- Various pains due to a stagnation of blood, rheumatic joint pain, impact injuries
- Constipation

- Skin infections, sores, carbuncles, boils

DOSAGE: 5–15 grams, decocted in water for an oral dose

NOTES: Angelica root stir-fried with wine increases its properties of promoting menstrual flow and increasing blood circulation.

Chinese Ginseng

ALTERNATE ENGLISH NAMES: Ginseng root, white ginseng

LATIN NAME: *Radix Ginseng*

PINYIN: Ren shen

FLAVOR: Sweet and slightly bitter

ESSENCE: Neutral

MERIDIANS: Enters the spleen, lung, and heart meridians

EFFECTS:

- Increases Qi, in this case, particularly "original" Qi, which forms the basis of kidney Qi
- Tones the spleen and lung
- Promotes production of blood and body fluids
- Calms the spirit
- Improves mental power

INDICATIONS:

- Depleted Qi or vital energy that can produce symptoms such as shortness of breath, listlessness, weak pulse; especially after a severe or prolonged illness
- A large loss of blood (such as that caused by childbirth, uterine bleeding, or traumatic injuries)
- Digestive disturbances such as loss of appetite, diarrhea
- Lung problems such as cough, shortness of breath
- Loss of body fluids (due to symptoms like spontaneous sweating, frequent urination, such as occurs in diabetes)
- Heart problems (with symptoms like palpitations)
- Insomnia, dream-disturbed sleep, irritability

DOSAGE: 5–10 grams, decocted alone with low heat and its decoction mixed with that of other herbs for an oral dose; 1–2 grams of ginseng root ground into powder and taken in capsule form 2–3 times per day; 15–30 grams for a large dosage.

Ginseng is the one herb that can increase Qi quickly. It can be used individually or in combination with foods or other herbs. For example, the following recipe is particularly good after surgery or after chemotherapy to help you increase Qi so you can recover faster.

Chicken and Ginseng

INGREDIENTS:
> Small baby or spring chicken
> 2 slices of fresh ginger
> Pinch of cinnamon
> 1 tablespoon cooking wine (optional)
> 1.5 ounces of ginseng
> Salt and pepper to taste

DIRECTIONS:
Start with a small baby or spring chicken. Add two slices of fresh ginger and a little bit of cinnamon. Add ginseng. If desired, add one tablespoon of cooking wine. Put all ingredients together in one pot. Cover with water to a depth of about two inches above the chicken. Bring to a boil; then let simmer for about an hour. Another way to cook this dish is to put all the ingredients in a crock pot, adding boiling water to two inches above the chicken. Simmer all day. When you're ready to eat, salt to taste. Eat this dish at least twice a week.

This dish can also be prepared with beef, lamb, or pork bone. If you're a vegetarian, cook the ginseng as above without meat and drink 1 cup of the liquid as a tea twice a day for at least a week.

PRECAUTIONS:

Ginseng should not be used in conjunction with black hellebore, trogopterus dung, and honey locust; tea and radish should be avoided during the time ginseng is used to avoid reducing its efficacy. TCM does *not* recommend taking ginseng for the common cold.

Poria

ALTERNATE ENGLISH NAMES: hoelen, tuckahoe
LATIN NAME: *Poria (Hoelen)*
PINYIN: Fu ling
FLAVOR: Sweet, tasteless in flavor
ESSENCE: Neutral
MERIDIANS: Enters heart, spleen, and kidney meridians
EFFECTS:

- Tones the spleen
- Diuretic (rids body of excess water, fluids; excretes dampness)
- Tranquilizes the spirit

INDICATIONS:

- Urinary tract problems such as painful or difficult urination, infections
- Edema (retention of water/fluids in the body)
- Excess phlegm, cough
- Digestive disturbances such as loss of appetite, loose stool
- Heart problems (which can result in symptoms like palpitations)
- Insomnia, fatigue, dizziness

DOSAGE: 10–15 grams, decocted in water for an oral dose

Red Sage Root

ALTERNATE ENGLISH NAMES: Red-rooted sage, salvia root

LATIN NAME: *Radix Salviae miltiorrhizae*

PINYIN: Dan shen

FLAVOR: Bitter

ESSENCE: Slightly cold

MERIDIANS: Enters the heart, pericardium, and liver meridians

EFFECTS:

- Increases blood circulation, nourishes (builds up) the blood (increases blood cells), relieves heat in the blood
- Calms the spirit

INDICATIONS:

- Menstrual problems such as PMS, painful periods, irregular periods; obstetrical problems
- Skin sores, carbuncles, boils
- Stomach and abdominal pain
- Masses in the abdomen
- Insomnia, irritability, palpitations

DOSAGE: 5–15 grams, decocted in water for an oral dose

PRECAUTIONS: Antagonistic to black hellebore rhizome.

White Atractylodes Rhizome

ALTERNATE ENGLISH NAMES: Atractylodes ovata rhizome

LATIN NAME: *Rhizoma Atractylodis macrocephalae*

PINYIN: Bai zhu

FLAVOR: Bitter and sweet

ESSENCE: Warm

MERIDIANS: Enters the heart, spleen, stomach, and triple warmer meridians

EFFECTS:

- Strengthens the spleen and stomach, balances the abdominal organs

- Diuretic (excretes dampness, especially from lower abdominal area)
- Prevents miscarriage

INDICATIONS:
- Digestive problems such as diarrhea, abdominal and epigastric distention, poor appetite
- Edema
- Restlessness, irritability
- Feeling of oppression in the chest
- Spontaneous sweating

DOSAGE: 5–10 grams, decocted in water for an oral dose; or ground into powder, or prepared in pill

Zedoary Rhizome

ALTERNATE ENGLISH NAMES: Zedoary
LATIN NAME: *Rhizoma Zedoariae*
PINYIN: E zhu
FLAVOR: Sour, sweet, slightly bitter
ESSENCE: Warm
MERIDIANS: Enters the lung, heart, and small intestine meridians

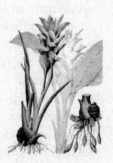

EFFECTS:
- Removes heat from body
- Invigorates flow of blood
- Detoxifies
- Reduces swelling, breaks up masses

INDICATIONS:
- Pain and distention in the regions of the heart and abdomen
- Stagnation of undigested food
- Menstrual difficulties, especially abnormal clotting
- Masses, tumors
- Sports injuries

DOSAGE: 5–10 grams, decocted in water for an oral dose

Licorice Root

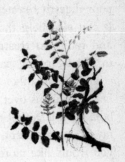

ALTERNATE ENGLISH NAMES: Licorice

LATIN NAME: *Radix Glycyrrhizae*

PINYIN: Gan cao

FLAVOR: Sweet

ESSENCE: Neutral

MERIDIANS: Enters the heart, lung, spleen, and stomach meridians

EFFECTS:

- Increases Qi or overall vital energy
- Tones the function of the spleen
- Relieves body of internal heat
- Detoxifies
- Relieves pain and spasm
- Harmonizes the properties of other herbs

INDICATIONS:

- Spleen functional problems involving poor appetite, diarrhea
- Cough, shortness of breath
- Skin infections such as sores, carbuncles, and boils
- Sore throat
- Food poisoning
- Stomachache, abdominal pain, muscular spasm and pain, spasm and pain in the extremities

DOSAGE: 2–10 grams, as the principal herb

There is a famous herbal formula that has been in use since the Sung Dynasty (960–1127 A.D.), which the Chinese call *Si Jun Zi Tang*. It combines licorice with ginseng, poria, and white atractolydos rhizome. Although it uses only four herbs, each one has a specific and unique healing role. This formula has been used for almost a thousand years to help increase the body's Qi and improve the function of the stomach and spleen.

This herbal formula is especially good for anyone with a

poor digestive system, loose stool, lack of appetite, and fatigue. It can also help those recovering from surgery, chemotherapy, and radiation treatment. This classical formula can be bought in tablet form at many Chinese herb stores. It forms the basis of a number of other classical Chinese herbal formulas that have helped millions over many centuries. Follow the directions on the box. (If you cannot find this formula locally, I have adapted it for my Western patients and it is called BCPP Herbal Master One. If you would like more information, please contact our foundation, whose address is in the back of this book.)

PRECAUTIONS: Licorice root is not to be used with kansui root, knoxia root, and genkwa flower; if licorice root is taken in large doses over a long period of time, it can possibly cause edema.

Notoginseng Root

ALTERNATE ENGLISH NAMES: Notoginseng, sanchi root

LATIN NAME(S): *Radix Notoginseng*

PINYIN: San qi

FLAVOR: Sweet and slightly bitter

ESSENCE: Warm

MERIDIANS: Enters the liver and stomach meridians

EFFECTS:

- The essence of notoginseng can increase blood flow (circulation) and also stop bleeding
- Helps the function of the heart and liver
- Increases Qi without the side effects associated with Chinese or American (or other types of) ginseng
- Relieves insomnia, palpitations
- Relieves pain
- Reduces swelling, inflammation, masses, tumors

INDICATIONS:

- Various types of internal bleeding (such as uterine bleed-

ing, coughing up of blood, blood in stool) and external bleeding (for example, due to traumatic injuries)
- Heart disease (such as angina pectoris)
- Sports injuries
- Breast masses, tumors, other types of masses and tumors

DOSAGE: 1–3 grams, ground into powder for swallowing (2,000–3,000 mg daily, powder in capsules); "proper amount" for external use

If you have blood stagnation, which can appear as clotting during your menstrual cycle, have blue marks on the side of your tongue, bruise easily, suffer from cardiovascular disease or varicose veins, or you've had a sports injury, notoginseng is one of the best herbs you can take.

Chicken with Notoginseng

INGREDIENTS:
Small baby or spring chicken
1 ounce notoginseng
2 teaspoons cooking wine
4 pieces of scallion
Salt

DIRECTIONS:
Combine notoginseng with cooking wine. Put four pieces of scallions with small baby or spring chicken. Cover with water to a depth of 2 inches above the chicken. Bring ingredients to a boil. Simmer for 1 hour. Salt to taste before eating.

Notoginseng Tea
You can now find notoginseng tea in some Chinese herb stores. It is an excellent blood tonic. Drink it daily to help prevent heart disease. (If you cannot find it locally, please contact our foundation for more information. You will find the address in the back of this book.)

Astragalus Root

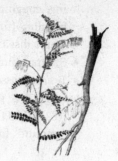

ALTERNATE ENGLISH NAMES: None

LATIN NAME: *Radix Astragali seu Hedysari*

PINYIN: Huang qi, Jin qi

FLAVOR: Sweet

ESSENCE: Warm

MERIDIANS: Enters the spleen and lung meridians

EFFECTS:

- Strengthens the immune system
- Tones and boosts Qi
- Diuretic
- Disperses swelling
- Detoxifies

INDICATIONS:

- Deficiency of Qi or vital energy, manifesting as symptoms of increased susceptibility to colds and flu, numbness in the extremities, spontaneous sweating, bleeding from uterus, blood in stool
- Spleen function problems (which can involve symptoms such as poor appetite, loose stool, lethargy)
- Prolapse of organs
- Skin problems/infections such as sores, carbuncles, boils
- Diabetes

DOSAGE: 10–15 grams, 30–60 grams for a large dosage, decocted in water for an oral dose

Astragalus Tonic

Many Chinese herb stores now have a tonic with astragalus. This tonic is particularly good for those with chronic fatigue or after surgery, chemotherapy and radiation.

Hawthorn Berry

ALTERNATE ENGLISH NAMES: Crataegus fruit, redhaw fruit
LATIN NAME: *Fructus Crataegi*
PINYIN: Shan zha
FLAVOR: Sour and sweet
ESSENCE: Slightly warm
MERIDIANS: Enters the spleen, stomach, and liver meridians
EFFECTS:

- Improves digestion
- Disperses and removes stagnant food
- Increases blood circulation, removes blood stagnation
- Expels tapeworm

INDICATIONS:

- Indigestion and retention of food (due to improper diet of too much greasy food and/or meat), symptoms of loss of appetite, abdominal distention, abdominal pain, diarrhea
- Masses, tumors (breast masses and/or tumors)
- Heart disease (angina pectoris, hypertension)
- Postpartum difficulties (pain, abnormal flow of lochia)

DOSAGE: 10–15 grams, 30–60 grams for a large dosage, decocted in water for an oral dose

Psoralea Fruit

ALTERNATE ENGLISH NAMES: None
LATIN NAME: *Fructus Psoraleae*
PINYIN: Bu gu zhi
FLAVOR: Pungent and bitter
ESSENCE: Warm
MERIDIANS: Enters the spleen and kidney meridians
EFFECTS:

- Helps kidney function

INDICATIONS:

- Lumbago
- Frequent urination

- Pain in the loins and knees (of a cold type)
- Cough, shortness of breath

DOSAGE: 5–10 grams, decocted in water for an oral dose, or used in pills or powder form

Dolichos Seed

ALTERNATE ENGLISH NAMES: Lablab seed
LATIN NAME: *Semen Dolichoris seu Lablab*
PINYIN: Bian dou
FLAVOR: Sweet
ESSENCE: Slightly warm
MERIDIANS: Enters the spleen and stomach meridians
EFFECTS:

- Strengthens Qi
- Balances digestive organs
- Relieves damp/heat in the body

INDICATIONS:

- Vomiting, diarrhea related to damp/heat climatic conditions
- Thirst, increased fluid intake, frequent urination, diabetes
- Poor appetite
- Vaginal discharge (both red and white)

DOSAGE: 5–12 grams, decocted in water for a daily dose

Lily Bulb

ALTERNATE ENGLISH NAMES: None
LATIN NAME: *Bulbus Lilii*
PINYIN: Bai he
FLAVOR: Sweet and slightly bitter
ESSENCE: Slightly cold
MERIDIANS: Enters the lung and heart meridians
EFFECTS:

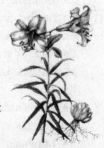

- Nourishes the lung, moistens the lung, arrests cough

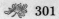

- Balances heart function, clears "fire" in the heart to quiet the spirit
- Gets rid of excess water in the body

INDICATIONS:

- Cough due to dryness of the lung, tubercular cough with sputum with blood
- Fever conditions, especially lingering fever
- Insomnia, clouded thinking
- Heart palpitations, especially stimulated by strong emotions
- Edema

DOSAGE: 10–30 grams, decocted in water for an oral dose

Safflower

ALTERNATE ENGLISH NAMES: Carthamus flower

LATIN NAME: *Flos Carthami*

PINYIN: Hong hua

FLAVOR: Pungent

ESSENCE: Warm

MERIDIANS: Enters the heart and liver meridians

EFFECTS:

- Increases blood circulation
- Eliminates blood stagnation
- Normalizes menstruation
- Breaks up masses
- Helps reduce body pains caused by stagnation of blood

INDICATIONS:

- Menstrual difficulties, including PMS, irregular periods, painful periods, absence of periods, "scanty" periods
- Postpartum pain, pain in lower abdomen
- Pain in the chest, hypochondrium (due to stagnation of blood)
- Masses in breast, masses in abdomen
- Sports injuries (impact injuries)

DOSAGE: 3–10 grams, decocted in water for an oral dose
PRECAUTIONS:

Safflower should not be prescribed for pregnant women and women with profuse menstruation.

White Peony Root

ALTERNATE ENGLISH NAMES: None

LATIN NAME: *Radix Paeoniae alba*

PINYIN: Bai shao yao

FLAVOR: Bitter and sour

ESSENCE: Slightly cold

MERIDIANS: Enters the liver and spleen meridians

EFFECTS:

- Nourishes the blood
- Regulates menstruation
- Nourishes the liver, balances liver function
- Reinforces yin with an astringent action to stop bleeding

INDICATIONS:

- Irregular menstruation, PMS, uterine bleeding, vaginal discharge
- Spontaneous sweating, night sweating
- Pain in the hypochondrium, stomach, and abdomen
- Vertigo, some types of headache

DOSAGE: 5–10 grams, 15–30 grams (large dosage), decocted in water for an oral dose

Germinated Barley

ALTERNATE ENGLISH NAMES: Dried barley sprout, malt

LATIN NAME: *Fructus Hordei germinates*

PINYIN: Mai ya

FLAVOR: Sweet and mild

ESSENCE: Neutral

MERIDIANS: Enters the stomach, spleen, and liver meridians

EFFECTS:
- Tones the digestive system
- Stops milk production in lactating women
- Helps liver function smoothly

INDICATIONS:
- Digestive system problems (for example, lactose and/or wheat intolerance, poor appetite, indigestion, food retention)
- Breast pain (a distending pain), to stop milk secretion

DOSAGE: 30–130 grams, decocted in water for an oral dose

The following recipe is very good for anyone who wants to keep their stomach function strong. It is also good for individuals who already have a digestive system problem, PMS, breast tenderness, or wheat or milk allergies. In my opinion, germinated barley offers much more benefit than wheatgrass. Use this herb as a tea or as a breakfast cereal.

Germinated Barley Recipes

Germinated barley may be difficult to find, but here's a simple way you can make your own. Buy a bag of organic barley. Soak in water overnight. Then strain the water and spread the barley evenly about 1 inch thick in an aluminum pan. Cover with a wet towel and keep in a warm place. Spray with water twice a day. Based on your room temperature, it should take about two days to germinate or sprout. When the sprouts reach about 1 inch in length, the barley is ready to be dried for use. One way to dry them is to put them in a slow oven under 200 degrees. Do not use high heat that will destroy the healing benefits of the barley. After drying, store in an airtight container.

Germinated Barley Tea

INGREDIENTS:

    2 handfuls (around 6 grams) germinated barley
    1–2 pieces fresh ginger
    2 slices tangerine peels

DIRECTIONS:

Take germinated barley, add fresh ginger, and tangerine peels, if available. Put in a pot and cover with 1 quart of water. Bring to a boil; then simmer for about twenty minutes. Strain this mixture and drink the water as a tea.

Germinated Barley Cereal

Another way to use germinated barley is to soak it overnight, then put it in a blender. Follow the above recipe until the boiling stage. Now you have an oatmeal-like mixture that you can eat for breakfast. You can add sesame seeds, peanuts, walnuts, or any other kind of nuts to enhance the flavor and healing benefits. Sweeten with honey and add cinnamon to taste.

PRECAUTIONS: Germinated barley should not be used by women who are breastfeeding.

Cinnamon Bark

    ALTERNATE ENGLISH NAME: None
    LATIN NAME: *Cortex Cinnamomi*
    PINYIN: Rou gui
    FLAVOR: Pungent and sweet
    ESSENCE: Hot
    MERIDIANS: Enters the kidney, spleen, liver, and heart
        meridians
    EFFECTS:

    • Helps kidney function

- Gets rid of cold conditions in the body
- Relieves pain
- Warms up and promotes flow of Qi through the meridians

INDICATIONS:

- Cold conditions such as cold limbs, feelings of aversion to cold
- Frequent urination
- Various pains (such as knee pain, lumbago)
- Gastric and abdominal pain, poor appetite, loose stool
- Menstrual problems such as painful periods, absence of periods, abnormal clotting
- Skin sores, abscesses, carbuncles, boils

DOSAGE: 2–5 grams, decocted later than other drugs when prepared for a decoction; 1–2 grams ground into a powder for an infusion taken orally

Corn Silk

ALTERNATE ENGLISH NAME: Zea, Maydis Stigmata

LATIN NAME: *Stigma maydis*

PINYIN: Yu mi xu

FLAVOR: Sweet

ESSENCE: Neutral

MERIDIANS: Enters the liver, gallbladder, stomach, and urinary bladder meridians

EFFECTS:

- Relieves water, dampness, and heat in the body
- Helps the gallbladder to pass stones (classically, in traditional Chinese medicine, corn silk has been prescribed for kidney stones and diabetes in addition to gallstones)
- Helps digestive system function well, particularly stomach and liver problems

INDICATIONS:

- Edema and swelling in the body
- Excess internal heat

- Gallstones
- Digestive disturbances such as diarrhea, belching, nausea

DOSAGE: 30–150 grams, decocted in water for an oral dose

Corn Silk Tea

Save the silk from ears of corn and dry it. Take a handful of corn silk (about 20 grams) and boil in 3 cups of water until the liquid has been reduced by half. Drink tea while it is hot. Drink twice a day.

Prunella

ALTERNATE ENGLISH NAMES: Self-heal, heal-all
LATIN NAME: *Spica Prunellae*
PINYIN: Xia ku cao
FLAVOR: Bitter, acrid
ESSENCE: Cold
MERIDIANS: Enters the liver and gallbladder meridians
EFFECTS:
- Helps the liver to function smoothly
- Breaks up lumps and masses

INDICATIONS:
- Lumps, masses, tumors in the body
- Goiter (swelling of the thyroid gland)
- Mammary abscess
- Excess tearing of the eyes and aversion to light, eyeball pain (especially at night)
- Sinew and bone pain
- Pulmonary tuberculosis
- Acute icteric (jaundice) infectious hepatitis
- Uterine bleeding

DOSAGE: 3–10 grams, decocted in water for an oral dose

Prunella Tea

Prunella tea is good for reducing tumors and helping skin problems. You can buy this at most Chinese herb stores. Put 2 ounces of the herb in 2 quarts of water. Bring to a boil. Let simmer for about thirty minutes. Drink this tea once or twice a day as part of your daily self-healing regimen.

Prunella and Oldenlandia Tea

These two herbs in combination have been used effectively by many TCM doctors to treat cancer and tumors. If you already have cancer, you can combine 1 ounce of prunella with 1 ounce of oldenlandia (see below) to make a tea that can be very useful during chemotherapy and radiation.

Oldenlandia

ALTERNATE ENGLISH NAMES: None
LATIN NAME: *Herba Oldenlandia diffusa*
PINYIN: Bai hua she she cao
FLAVOR: Bitter and sweet
ESSENCE: Cold
MERIDIANS: Enters the stomach, large intestine, and small intestine meridians
EFFECTS:
- Relieves/reduces heat in the body
- Relieves damp conditions internally
- Shrinks masses and tumors
- Detoxifies internal poisons (Oldenlandia has been used classically in traditional Chinese medicine both internally and externally to treat poisons, e.g., snakebite)

INDICATIONS:
- Cancer

- Various forms of poisoning or conditions where toxins have built up in the body
- Masses, tumors

DOSAGE: 15–60 grams, decocted in water for an oral dose

Oldenlandia Tea

Many Chinese herb stores carry Oldenlandia in powdered form, from which you can make a tea. (If you cannot find this herb locally, please contact our foundation for more information. You'll find the address at the back of this book.)

Chinese Yam Rhizome

ALTERNATE ENGLISH NAMES: Dioscorea rhizome
LATIN NAME: *Rhizoma Dioscoreae*
PINYIN: Shan yao, Huai shan yao
FLAVOR: Sweet
ESSENCE: Neutral
MERIDIANS: Enters the spleen, lung, and kidney meridians
EFFECTS:

- Strengthens the kidney
- Improves the function of the spleen and stomach
- Promotes production of body fluids to nourish the lung

INDICATIONS:

- Deficiency of the kidney (which can manifest in symptoms such as frequent urination, vaginal discharge)
- Digestive problems such as poor appetite, loose stool or diarrhea
- Cough, shortness of breath
- Diabetes, loss of body fluids, thirst

DOSAGE: 10–30 grams, large dosage 60–250 grams, decocted in water for an oral dose; or ground into powder for an oral administration: 6–10 grams each time

PRECAUTIONS: Do not use in cases of abdominal distention due to excessive dampness or food stagnancy.

Coix Seed

ALTERNATE ENGLISH NAMES: Job's tears seed

LATIN NAME: *Semen Coicis*

PINYIN: Yi ren mi, Yi mi ren

FLAVOR: Bland and sweet

ESSENCE: Cold

MERIDIANS: Enters the spleen, lung and kidney meridians

EFFECTS:

- Strengthens the spleen
- Strengthens the lung
- Eliminates dampness from the body
- Relieves the body of excess internal heat

INDICATIONS:

- Obstruction of meridians, particularly by dampness
- Arthritic pain (due to dampness), muscular spasm in the limbs
- Edema
- Diarrhea
- Weakness of the lungs
- Vaginal discharge

DOSAGE: 10–30 grams, decocted in water for an oral dose

Coix Seed Breakfast Dish

This herb is particularly good for preventing cancer. It can help strengthen your digestive system and help rid the body of edema, or excess water. It is also useful for helping reduce arthritis pain. You can cook this as a breakfast dish.

INGREDIENTS:

> Take 1 cup of Coix seed, add 1 cup of lotus seed, and 1 cup of Chinese red dates. You can also add raw peanuts to this dish. Put ingredients in a pot and add 2 quarts of water. Bring to a boil and then simmer for about forty minutes until the mixture cooks down. You can sweeten to taste with honey or brown sugar. This dish makes enough for about five days. You can cook it ahead of time and reheat each morning. You can add more water, soy or regular milk, if you prefer a thinner consistency.

PRECAUTIONS: Use with care during pregnancy.

Ginkgo Leaf

ALTERNATE ENGLISH NAMES: Ginkgo leaf

LATIN NAME: *Folium Ginkgo*

PINYIN: Bae guo ye

FLAVOR: Sweet and slightly bitter

ESSENCE: Neutral

MERIDIANS: Enters the lung and stomach meridians

EFFECTS:

- Relieves pain
- Nourishes lung, relieves cough
- Promotes general circulation
- Helps heart disease

INDICATIONS:

- High cholesterol, high blood pressure, palpitations
- Coughs (any kind of cough)

DOSAGE: 3–6 grams, decocted in water; 500–1000 mg, powdered form in capsule for a daily dose

American Ginseng

ALTERNATE ENGLISH NAMES: Man's health, tartar root, five fingers

LATIN NAME: *Radix Panacis Quinquefolii*

PINYIN: Xi yang shen

FLAVOR: Sweet and slightly bitter
ESSENCE: Neutral
MERIDIANS: Enters the heart, lung, and kidney meridians
EFFECTS:

- Tones Qi and blood
- Relieves heat in body
- Promotes production of body fluids

INDICATIONS:

- Lung problems, especially heat in lung, cough (all kinds)
- Loss of fluids and blood (i.e., during chemotherapy, radiation, after surgery)
- Constipation

DOSAGE: 500–1000 mg powder in capsule form for daily use

Lycium Berry

ALTERNATE ENGLISH NAMES: Wolfberry, Chinese matrimony vine berry
LATIN NAME: *Fructus Lycii*
PINYIN: Gou qi zi
FLAVOR: Sweet
ESSENCE: Neutral
MERIDIANS: Enters the liver, kidney, and lung meridians
EFFECTS:

- Strengthens the kidney, replenishes the vital essence of kidney
- Nourishes the liver
- Improves vision
- Moistens and nourishes the lung

INDICATIONS:

- Deficiency in function of kidney (sometimes manifesting as weakness, particularly in the thighs and legs, sore lower back, soreness in knees)
- Blurred vision
- Dizziness

- Lung problems, particularly cough and a condition of dryness in the lung

DOSAGE: 5–10 grams, decocted in water for an oral dose

Motherwort

ALTERNATE ENGLISH NAMES: Chinese motherwort, leonurus

LATIN NAME: *Herba Leonuri*

PINYIN: Yi mu cao

FLAVOR: Pungent and bitter

ESSENCE: Slightly cold

MERIDIANS: Enters the heart, liver, and urinary bladder meridians

EFFECTS:

- Diuretic
- Increases blood circulation, removes blood stagnation
- Clears internal heat from body
- Detoxifies
- Helps heart

INDICATIONS:

- Edema, difficulty in urinating
- Irregular or stagnant menstruation, absence of menstruation
- Postpartum abdominal pain
- Distending pain in lower abdomen
- Sports injuries, traumatic injuries with pain and swelling
- Skin sores, infections
- Heart disease such as angina pectoris

DOSAGE: 10–15 grams decocted in water for oral dose; for inducing diuresis to treat edema, the large dosage can be 30–60 grams

NOTE: Used externally on skin sores, infections

CHAPTER 18

How You Can Access Seven Secret Healing Gates to Achieve Maximum Health Benefits

*I*n the human body, there are many special acupoints or "healing gates" that can help your organs communicate with each other harmoniously. Like the junction where several major highways come together, these points let a maximum amount of Qi or energy flow through. Some points are stronger than others and can help you accumulate more healing Qi. How to locate some of these points and apply their healing benefits for specific problems is knowledge that is not necessarily found in TCM medical texts. Rather, it's information passed over many generations from master to student. I have been fortunate enough to receive this kind of high-level medical knowledge from several of my masters. It is my privilege to share this gift with you.

If you do not have breast cancer, using acupuncture or massage daily on these points can help you reduce a range of symptoms that TCM considers early warning signals of critical imbalances and Qi or energy dysfunctions. If you have breast cancer, using acupressure or massage daily on these points or in these areas can help your body recover more quickly from chemotherapy, radiation, or side effects from cancer treatments. Incorporating acupressure into your daily routine can also help your organs function in harmony. When you accomplish this, you can gain more strength to go through breast cancer treatments that compromise the immune system. Daily acupressure or massage can also help fight cancer's negative energy pattern. Continuing this routine over time can help prevent cancer from recurring.

Most of these healing gates are bilateral or located on each side of your body. You can massage individual points or a combination. I recommend that you massage each one for at least five minutes a day for maximum effect. Following are seven special healing gates that you can work with.

1. This first important healing gate can help your body generate Qi to fight breast cancer. The point is located at the center of the bottom of each of your feet. You can massage this point with your thumb, or a tennis ball, or whatever you have on hand that helps stimulate it. This point can strengthen your Qi foundation. If you already have breast cancer, you can use moxibustion (see page 165) to warm this point: cut a thin slice of fresh ginger about the size of a quarter, place it over this point, and use the heat of moxibustion to penetrate the ginger and drive its essence into this point. (Smokeless moxibustion

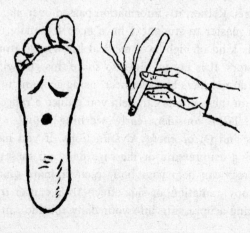

sticks of herbs can be found at most Chinese herb stores, acupuncture medical supply companies, and Western natural food stores.) Do this for about five minutes on the bottom of each foot.

2. The second most important healing gate is located about the width of four fingers directly below your belly button. This point can also generate extra Qi for healing purposes and longevity. Massage this point gently in small circles in both directions. For those without breast cancer, this point can help relieve menstrual cramps; help infertility; rebalance any kind of hormone problems, and help alleviate many kinds of female problems. If you already have breast cancer and are undergoing chemotherapy or radiation, use ginger and moxibustion in the same way described above.

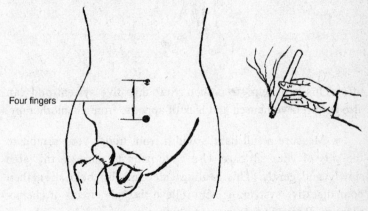

Four fingers

3. From under your breastbone or sternum to above your belly button, there is an area that you can massage gently to generate more Qi for healing. Put one hand on top of the other with your palms on this area. Slowly and gently make a circle clockwise five times; reverse direction and make a circle counterclockwise five times. Continue this routine for about five min-

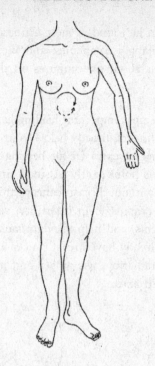

utes. This can help strengthen your digestive system and can also help relieve nausea and lack of appetite from chemotherapy.

4. Measure a full hand's width from under your armpit to the side of your rib cage. Use your palm to massage this area slowly and gently. This healing gate can also help strengthen your digestive system, or help relieve the side effects of chemotherapy. Remember to massage both sides.

5. Where the two bones of the thumb and the index finger meet, there is another healing gate. It is located at the bottom of the index finger bone in the "V" shape. Using your opposite thumb, press or massage this point in a circle. After massaging this point, continue to gently massage the entire index finger bone toward the first knuckle of the index finger. This is a

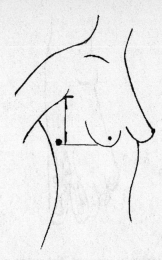

technique you can practice anywhere, any time. This helps stimulate the Qi of the stomach, large intestine, and lung so that these organs begin to work in harmony as they are supposed to do.

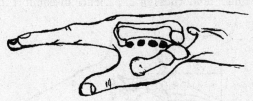

6. Likewise, on the top of the foot, there is another healing gate where the big toe bone meets the second toe bone. Massage and press this spot with your thumb. Again, using your thumb, slide your finger continuously toward the tip of your second toe. You may feel some pain or discomfort; this means you are on the right spot and unblocking Qi stagnation in your liver meridian. This is a very important healing gate. (Remember that the liver is the most important organ for women's health.) The degree of pain will tell you how badly affected your liver func-

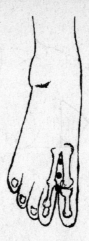

tion is. The more stressed you are, the more pain you will have. Try to massage this area frequently.

7. There is a healing gate in the middle of the top of each of your shoulders. Use your thumb or finger to locate this point. You may find a tenderness or experience discomfort in a certain

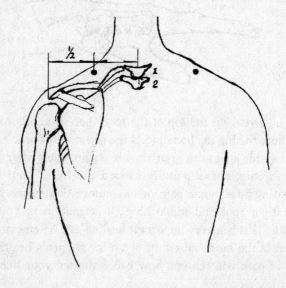

area. This means you have found the right spot. Massaging both sides can help you relieve Qi blockages in your neck and shoulders. It can also help relieve a Qi blockage in your breast area. Women with breast masses should press more deeply.

Conclusion

As I hope you've learned, TCM can help you with many different stages of your health problems. The very best part of TCM is prevention. Remember that each and every one of you reading this book is born with the ability to heal yourself. As we know, real prevention means taking charge of your own health and healing. If you have minor health problems, tackle them immediately. Don't wait until they become chronic or severe. Don't be like the warrior in the *Nei Jing* who sharpens his sword in the middle of battle. You might be too late! Be as aggressive as you need to be to help yourself heal. Always take your symptoms seriously. Do not let anyone tell you "you're making a mountain out of a molehill."

If you have breast cancer or any other deep health problem, don't think that just because you've had surgery or been through chemotherapy and radiation, that you can resume your old ways. You now must work at least twice as hard to stay as healthy as you used to be. Remember that TCM believes it is your old lifestyle that allowed disease or illness to occur in the first place. TCM says this not to blame you, but to help you understand that the problem has occurred because your internal

Qi has become unbalanced and therefore hospitable to negative energy. Because the problem is internal, the key to fixing it is also internal. Once you understand this, you can then apply this ancient knowledge to create a strong energy field that can defeat any kind of cancer and prevent it from taking hold in your body.

Many of my patients and students have urged me to write this book. They believe that Western women with breast cancer or breast cancer recurrence, as well as those who want to remain healthy and prevent this disease, would welcome the opportunity to learn how to take responsibility for their own health and healing.

It has been my privilege to share this wisdom with you. I hope you've learned a lot about yourself and how your body really works by reading this book. I also hope that you will use the time-tested TCM principles, theories and techniques that are outlined here every day to help you unlock your own healing ability.

Remember, the power to heal yourself is always yours.

Traditional Chinese Medicine Evaluation Form for Charting Your Healing Progress

To follow is your TCM self-healing evaluation form. You do have the power to heal yourself and keeping track of your healing progress can give you great hope and strength. Make extra copies for each week you plan to work with the information in this book. The questions on the form are based on TCM diagnosis. Fill it out before you begin, so that you can track your progress as your Qi becomes stronger and your body's organs return to a more balanced state. You should experience benefits in the areas you've noted as a health problem. This is a good sign that you have begun to unblock Qi in critical meridians and are restoring harmony to key organs. As your symptoms improve, feel this self-healing power working. You have used your own healing ability to put yourself on the road to well-being.

If you are interested in ordering the Breast Cancer Prevention Project (BCPP) Herbal Master formulas and teas that I have developed for my own patients, please contact our foundation for more information.

TCM PERSONAL SELF-HEALING EVALUATION FORM

This form may be used to monitor your self-healing progress as you follow the Breast Cancer Prevention Project nine-point guide.

The following questions are used by TCM practitioners to understand the condition of the functions of the major organs. Use the following to identify the current condition of the function of your major organs. This will be your baseline. Decide how you wish to evaluate them. Assess the degree that each of these symptoms affects you on a daily, weekly, or monthly basis. Incorporate the steps of our nine-point self-healing guide into your daily life and monitor your progress.

PLEASE CIRCLE THE APPROPRIATE ANSWER OR FILL IN THE BLANKS WHEN APPLICABLE

Have you been troubled by the following symptoms?

1. Fatigue	Y/N	10. Loss of appetite	Y/N	19. Depression	Y/N
2. Dizziness	Y/N	11. Abdominal distention	Y/N	20. Nightmares	Y/N
3. Palpitations	Y/N	12. Headache	Y/N	21. Nervousness	Y/N
4. Hot flashes	Y/N	13. Stomachache	Y/N	22. Angry moods	Y/N
5. Night sweats	Y/N	14. Diarrhea	Y/N	23. Worrying	Y/N
6. Shortness of breath	Y/N	15. Constipation	Y/N	24. Loss of sexual interest	Y/N
7. Chest pain	Y/N	16. Skin rash	Y/N	25. Forgetting information	Y/N
8. Back pain	Y/N	17. Dry mouth	Y/N	26. Frequent urination	Y/N
9. Muscle tension	Y/N	18. Insomnia	Y/N	27. Cold hands and feet	Y/N

Your Menstrual History:

1. First year menstrual cycle started ____

2. Menstrual Cramps ____ none ____ before ____ during ____ after

3. Menstrual Disorders ____ early ____ late ____ irregular ____ short ____ long cycle

4. Other conditions before cycle ____ diarrhea ____ constipation ____ headache ____ bloating

5. Vaginal discharge ____ none ____ white ____ yellow ____ heavy

6. Flow (quantity) ____ no. of days ____ light ____ heavy ____ clotting ____ small ____ large

7. Color of blood ____ light ____ dark

Breast Cancer History:

1. Do you have a family history of breast cancer? Y/N Who? _____

2. Have you ever had a breast mass or tumor? Y/N When? _____ Location? _____ left _____ right

3. Have you been diagnosed with breast cancer? Y/N Stages _____ I _____ II _____ III _____ IV
   When _____? Location? _____ left breast _____ right breast _____

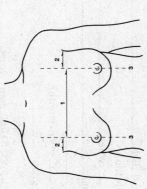

1. Related to kidney and liver
2. Related to liver and stomach
3. Related to stomach

4. What kind of treatments have you undergone? _____

5. Have you had chemotherapy? Y/N How long? _____ Radiation? Y/N How long? _____

6. Are you taking any anti-estrogenic agents? Y/N How long? _____ Which one(s)? _____

7. Have you had side effects from anti-estrogenic treatment? Y/N

8. Please list: _____

_____

_____

Other Physical Conditions

1. ____ heart disease ____ heart attack ____ arrhythmias ____ angina ____ medication

2. ____ allergies ____ food ____ other ____ fall ____ spring ____ all year

3. ____ high blood pressure ____ how long ____ special diet ____ medication

4. ____ diabetes ____ how long ____ special diet ____ medication

5. ____ high cholesterol ____ special medication

6. ____ any organs removed ____ when ____ which one(s)

7. ____ any other major medical problems? ____

8. Are you pregnant? ____ no ____ yes ____ what month?

9. How many times have you been pregnant? ____

10. Have you ever breast fed? Y/N

11. Have you ever used birth control pills? Y/N How many years? ____

Resource List

*A*CCORDING to the National Acupuncture Foundation, acupuncture and Oriental Medicine are among the fastest growing healthcare professions in the United States. Today, there are 13,000 practicing acupuncturists and Americans are making between 9 and 12 million visits yearly. There are also 68 schools of traditional Chinese medicine located in the U.S. The list of organizations below can provide information on those who provide acupuncture or TCM services.

American Association of Oriental Medicine
433 Front Street
Catasaqua, PA 18032
(P) 610-266-1433
(Q) 610-264-2768
E-mail: aaom.org

American Foundation of Traditional Chinese Medicine
505 Beach Street
San Francisco, CA 94133
(P) 415-776-0502

American Holistic Health Association
PO Box 17400
Anaheim, CA 92817-7400
(P) 714-779-6152
E-mail: www.ahha.org

American Holistic Medical Association (AHMA)
6728 Old McLean Village Drive
McLean, VA 22101
(P) 703-556-9728

American Oriental Bodywork Therapy Association
1010 Haddonfield Berlin Road #408
Voorhees, NJ 08403
(P) 609-782-1616
E-mail: www.abmp.com

Association of Holistic Healing Centers
Margaret Irby, Ph.D.
PO Box 2367
Carefree, AZ 85377
(P) 602-488-5502
(F) 602-588-1371
E-mail: ahhcirby@aol.com

Council of Colleges of Acupuncture and Oriental Medicine
1010 Wayne Avenue, Suite 1270
Silver Spring, MD 20910
(P) 301-608-9175

National Acupuncture and Oriental Medicine Alliance
1437 Starr Road, S.E.
Olalla, WA 98359
(P) 253-851-6896
(F) 253-851-6883
E-mail: www.acuall.org.

Traditional Acupuncture Institute
American City Building, 10227
Wincopin Circle, Suite 100
Columbia, MD 21044
(P) 301-596-6006

Acknowledgments

I would like to extend my deepest appreciation and thanks to my masters, particularly Professor Xi-hua Xu, who continues to open up new worlds of healing knowledge to me. I would like to thank my patients, who have taught me many things, not the least of which is patience. In particular, I would like to thank those special patients who were kind enough to encourage this effort and generous enough to share their insights with me.

I would like to thank all my Qigong students and let them know how much their good wishes and continued support and care mean to me. For all their help and dedication to making the world of traditional Chinese medicine interesting and accessible to people in the West, I would like to thank Heather Allen, Louise DiBello, Ellasara Kling, and Kristen Park. Each has helped this effort in a special way; all have been instrumental in bringing the Center's work to a new level. Karen Schulz has continually been there when we needed her time, attention and excellent graphics work. Her willingness to explore new directions and give us good advice with good humor is much appreciated. Debra Bernath deserves a special thanks for lending her talents in the area of art work. I would like to acknowledge Jaime Phillips for his excellent photography of a challenging assignment and the Eddy Foundation for generously underwriting this need.

Kostas Vaxevaneris and Susan Slack of Omega Design Communications deserve special recognition for their long hours of work and their dedication to perfection, which went above and beyond at every stage in creating an earlier version of this work. Thank you also to the talented professionals at Ruder Finn, Inc., especially Senior Video Producer Ed Goldstein who made a major contribution with his work on our video.

Ellen and I continue to marvel at the role fate has played in meeting our extraordinary agent Barbara Lowenstein of Lowenstein & Associates, and her interest in our work. For her enthusiasm for our initial manuscript, for nurturing it, and for believing in the power of this work, we thank you. Thank you also for working with us at every opportunity to make this effort the best that it can be. For walking us through the amazing creative process of delivering a real live book, we're most grateful to our special editor, Ann McKay Thoroman of Avon Books. Her gentle yet probing questions, natural inquisitiveness, and commitment to seeing this unique manuscript published are deeply appreciated. Her reassurances and encouragement were essential to sustaining our confidence in thinking we could write such a comprehensive work.

Finally, I would like to thank my writing partner Ellen Schaplowsky for spending so many hours on this book, for worrying about the details—large and small—and for helping me bring this ancient knowledge to life. Without her dedication, deep understanding, and determination to finding the right words and phrases to help make TCM accessible to a Western audience, this book would not have seen the light as soon nor as well. Without her help, I could not have achieved my mission of sharing this knowledge with you. She has used her special gift to capture my words and concepts about TCM and develop them into a language that everyone can understand and hopefully use. Her contribution to this work has been invaluable.

About Nan Lu, O.M.D., L.Ac.

*T*HE Breast Cancer Prevention Project was founded and developed by Nan Lu, O.M.D., L.Ac. Dr. Lu is also president of the Traditional Chinese Medicine Foundation and founding director of the American Taoist Healing Center, Inc., of New York and New Jersey. The Center is the only facility of its kind dedicated to teaching *Wu Ming* Qigong in the United States. Dr. Lu is a classically trained doctor of TCM and a New York State licensed acupuncturist. His Foundation is dedicated to serving as the source for authentic information on Taoist Qigong and TCM. Its mission is to build bridges of understanding between East and West in the areas of TCM, natural healing, and internal martial arts.

Dr. Lu began his training in China at an early age in Taoist Qigong, TCM, and internal martial arts. Studying with several well-known, well-respected masters and doctors, he received special keys of understanding and the true essence of these ancient healing and internal martial arts. The unique healing knowledge Dr. Lu has acquired cannot be found in medical textbooks. His extensive training is the kind that ancient doctors of TCM were expected to have so that they could understand the fundamental theory of TCM—how Qi moves through the body. As a Qigong master and international martial arts champion, Dr. Lu has refined his energy practice to a very high level.

An extraordinary martial artist, Dr. Lu has won many top honors. In the fall of 1997, he competed in Argentina in the Sixth International World Cup Championship where he was named one of the top ten Taiji masters in the world. He has authored many columns for internal martial arts publications including *Pa Kua Chang* Journal, *Wushu Kung Fu,* and *Inside Kung Fu* magazines.

He is a member of the advisory group of participants for Columbia University's Center for Complementary & Alternative Medicine Research in Women's Health in a landmark study of Chinese herbs. He is also a board director of the American Acupuncture Association, an advisory board member of the Transpersonal Psychology Association, the Hypoglycemia Support Foundation, and the USA Wushu Kungfu Federation. In New York, he works with SHARE, a major self-help organization for women with breast or ovarian cancer. Through SHARE, Dr. Lu teaches many of the *Wu Ming* Qigong movements to women with breast cancer to help them improve breast and ovarian health.

Dr. Lu holds a Doctorate in Oriental Medicine from Hubei College of Traditional Chinese Medicine, China, and a Master of Science degree from City University of New York (CUNY), Herbert Lehman College. He has authored numerous articles on TCM and Taoist Qigong. With his "Eastern Outlook" column for *Natural Way,* Dr. Lu was the first-ever columnist on TCM for a national health magazine. His practice includes the use of many herbal supplements based on ancient traditional Chinese formulas that he has developed and adapted for his Western patients. He has also developed a TCM skin care treatment line based on TCM principles. Dr. Lu has lectured extensively on TCM, Qigong, and self-healing in China, the United States, and England.

About Ellen Schaplowsky

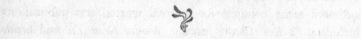

ELLEN Schaplowsky has more than 20 years of experience in marketing communications work for consumer products, and in reputation management and environmental marketing. She is an executive vice president of Ruder Finn, Inc., one of the world's largest independent public relations agencies, where she founded the company's "Marketing for the Environment" Group. The Group's mission is to help corporations, brand businesses, and nonprofit organizations communicate on complex issues so that practical solutions can be identified. As part of her work in this area, Ellen has served as a guest columnist for the *Earth Times*, the first global newspaper on issues of the environment and sustainability that emerged from the 1992 Earth Summit in Rio de Janeiro. She is also responsible for helping create and develop America's largest litter cleanup and recycling program that annually attracts several million volunteers. For thirteen years, this program was conducted jointly by GLAD® brand and Keep America Beautiful, Inc. It is regarded as one of the longest running partnerships in brand history.

During the early 1990s, Ellen was searching for an explanation and treatment for a complex of physical symptoms that no

Western doctor seemed able to pinpoint and treat. After a number of years, she was diagnosed as having an autoimmune condition. It was at about the same time that she was introduced to the concept of Qi or "energy" and met Nan Lu, O.M.D., L.Ac. Ellen became Dr. Lu's patient and began a journey that would bring her deeper and deeper into traditional Chinese medicine (TCM) and its approach to self-healing and wellness. Eventually, she began practicing *Wu Ming* Qigong under the guidance of Dr. Lu.

While a patient and student, Ellen began applying her marketing communications skills to help Dr. Lu achieve his mission of serving as the authentic source for information on traditional Chinese medicine and Taoist Qigong. At Dr. Lu's request, she became the Foundation's vice president. In 1996, she and Dr. Lu began collaborating on writing the first-ever column on TCM for a national health magazine, *Natural Way*. After more than two years of developing this column, they embarked on a more ambitious writing project, the first version of what would become *Traditional Chinese Medicine: A Woman's Guide to Healing from Breast Cancer*. This effort marks their first book in a series of TCM works to be published by Avon Books.

Ellen lives in Upper Montclair, New Jersey, and has a son, Ian, who lives in Boston.

About the Traditional Chinese Medicine World Foundation

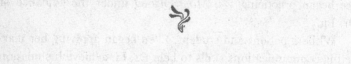

*T*HE Foundation is a nonprofit organization, founded by author Nan Lu, O.M.D., L.Ac. Its mission is to build bridges of understanding between the East and West through educational programs in Qigong, TCM, natural healing, and internal martial arts. It is dedicated to serving as the source for authentic information on TCM and Taoist Qigong.

The following programs and projects are conducted by the Foundation:

Traditional Chinese Medicine World, **The Newspaper of Authentic Health and Healing**

The Foundation publishes the first national newspaper on TCM to help educate Western health-seekers about this ancient medical system and how it can enhance their well-being.

The Breast Cancer Prevention Project

The Breast Cancer Prevention Project was launched in 1997. Its mission is to bring the ancient self-healing knowledge of TCM and its centuries-old experience with breast cancer to as many women as possible. Recently, the Foundation began the Tamoxifen Program as part of the Breast Cancer Prevention Project. This seven-session program uses TCM principles and theories to treat the root cause of the menopausal symptoms caused by the antiestrogenic agent tamoxifen. The Breast Cancer Prevention Project includes this book, *A Woman's Guide to Healing from Breast Cancer*; a companion video; outreach programs with organizations like SHARE, the New York self-help organization for women with breast or ovarian cancer; and a website at www.breastcancer.com.

Women's Health Including PMS and Menopause Programs

The Foundation conducts programming for women's health that includes a special six-week course to help alleviate the symptoms of menopause like hot flashes, night sweats, insomnia, and irritability. TCM has been treating menopausal symptoms for thousands of years by addressing their common root cause—unbalanced liver Qi and kidney deficiency. In fact, one famous herbal formula for hot flashes has been in use for centuries and is still used today in China.

Dragon's Way®

The Dragon's Way is the Foundation's successful self-healing program for weight loss and stress management. It addresses the underlying factors causing weight problems in a seven-session program. The Dragon's Way uses the best of TCM principles and theories to help individuals heal themselves and lose weight. It combines *Wu Ming* Meridian Therapy, a special eating for healing plan, and TCM herbal formulas for maximum health. To date, more than five hundred individuals have gone through the program with excellent results. Participants lose on average 12 pounds and 8 inches. Most important are the reductions in problems such as stress, cholesterol, and high blood pressure and the alleviation of other helath issues, including insomnia, food allergies, and stomach conditions, to name a few.

About the American Taoist
Healing Center, Inc.

❧

*T*HE American Taoist Healing Center, Inc. was founded and is also under the direction of Nan Lu, O.M.D., L.Ac. The Center is dedicated to serving as the source for authentic information and training on TCM and Taoist Qigong.

PROGRAMMING

TCM Treatment

Dr. Lu maintains a practice in New York City and Bloomfield, New Jersey. He uses Taoist Qigong, acupressure, acupuncture (in New York City), moxibustion, herbs and Chinese medical massage to treat a variety of conditions. Areas of specialty include: women's health, especially breast cancer, PMS, menopause, menstrual irregularities; chronic fatigue syndrome; arthritis; hayfever; allergies; tendinitis; and sports injuries, to name a few. The focus of his practice is on preventing illness and disease, as well as helping patients heal themselves.

Taoist *Wu Ming* Qigong

Wu Ming Qigong is the foundation of all programming at

the American Taoist Healing Center and Dr. Lu's medical practice. This unique self-healing energy system has never before been taught in the United States. It descends directly from the ancient Taoist masters Lao Tzu and Chuang Tzu. This special self-healing energy practice, which is easy to learn and produces results rapidly, helps students (and patients) connect their body, mind, spirit and emotions for maximum healing benefit. *Wu Ming* Qigong is taught in beginner and advanced levels.

Qigong Meridian Therapy (QMT)

The American Taoist Healing Center conducts training in Qigong Meridian Therapy (QMT) for therapists, which includes a grounding in the fundamentals of TCM and Taoist Qigong, as well as intensive training in special hand techniques for this medical treatment. QMT practitioners are certified jointly with the Center and Hubei College of TCM, Hubei, China. QMT practitioners have offered their services at a number of large firms and organizations, including Smith Barney, New York Department of Personnel, and the Mind/Body Medical Center of Morristown Hospital in New Jersey, among others.

PRODUCTS

The following products have been developed by Nan Lu O.M.D., L.Ac., and are based on the principles and theories of TCM.

   🦚 *Traditional Chinese Medicine—A Healing Guide For Breast Cancer*
—companion video with Nan Lu, O.M.D., L.Ac. teaching *Wu Ming* Meridian Therapy movements. Video also features a full twenty-minute practice session with Dr. Lu.

   🦚 All-Natural Herbal Food Supplements for a variety of health conditions, including:

—The Breast Cancer Prevention Project (BCPP) Herbal Master line of herbs and natural herbal teas.

❧ All-Natural Herbal Skin Treatment Products

—Acne Facial Masque: herbal masque that helps correct underlying cause of acne
—All Day/All Night Creme: stimulates meridians in the facial area and brings more nutrition into the face for a smoother, younger appearance
—Silk Face Masque: a special all-natural combination of TCM herbs that is blended with honey; helps pull toxins from the skin and creates smooth, fresh-looking appearance.

For more information, contact:
Traditional Chinese Medicine World Foundation
396 Broadway, Suite 501
New York, N.Y. 10013
Phone: 212-274-1079
www.tcmworld.org
www.breastcancer.com

Index